OSCE

A teaching manual for medical undergraduates

4th Edition

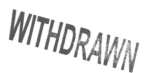

Ruth Bird
Simon Fleming
Helen Twohig
Ali Majeed

www.oscemanual.com

OSCE
A teaching manual for medical undergraduates

4th Edition

Ruth Bird
Simon Fleming
Helen Twohig
Ali Majeed

www.oscemanual.com

Published by:

A W Majeed
Cliffe Cottage
66 Ranmoor Road
Sheffield S10 3HJ

First Edition 2003
Second Edition 2003
Third Edition 2006
Fourth Edition 2008
Reprinted 2010
Reprinted 2012

ISBN 0-9545032-0-1

www.oscemanual.com

This book is dedicated to the memory of

Professor Alan Godfrey Johnson

Contents

Acknowledgements	vii
Background and Design of OSCEs	viii
How to use this book	xx
Abbreviations used	xxi
Gastrointestinal system	1
General gastrointestinal history	2
Presenting complaint - abdominal pain	4
Presenting complaint - dysphagia	7
Presenting complaint - dyspepsia	9
Presenting complaint - vomiting	10
Presenting complaint - jaundice	12
Presenting complaint - diarrhoea	14
Presenting complaint - constipation	16
Presenting complaint - rectal bleeding	18
Examination of the GI system	20
Digital Rectal Examination	25
Examination of a Groin Hernia	27
Examination of a patient with acute abdominal pain	29
Gastrointestinal Bleeding	32
Alcohol History	34
Cardiovascular system	36
General cardiovascular history	37
Presenting complaint - chest pain	39
Presenting complaint - palpitations	42
Presenting complaint - intermittent claudication	44
Examination of the cardiovascular system	46
Examination of the precordium	50
Peripheral vascular examination	54
Top Tips: Understanding ECGs	57
Tachycardias	64
Bradycardias	71
Respiratory system	77
General respiratory history	78
Presenting complaint - cough	80
Presenting complaint - shortness of breath	83
Examination of the respiratory system	85
Top Tips: Looking at Chest X-rays	89
Inhaler Technique	112
Peak Flow Measurement	113
Neurological system	114
General neurological history	115
Presenting complaint - headache and facial pain	118
Presenting complaint - sudden onset weakness	120
Presenting complaint - collapse	122
Examination of the cranial nerves	125

Examination of the lower limbs	130
Examination of the upper limbs	133
Cognitive state assessment	136
Top Tips: Neurological Examination	137
Musculoskeletal system	141
Presenting complaint - joint pain	142
Presenting complaint - back pain	145
Examination of the musculoskeletal system (GALS)	147
Examination of the hands	150
Examination of the hip	152
Examination of the knee	154
Examination of a patient with back pain	156
Endocrine system	159
General endocrine history	160
Suspected diabetes mellitus	164
Suspected thyroid dysfunction	166
Examination for hypothyroidism	168
Examination for thyrotoxicosis	169
Examination of a goitre	171
Examination of a diabetic foot	173
Genitourinary system	175
General urinary tract history	176
Presenting complaint - haematuria	179
Sexual medical history	181
Presenting complaint - vaginal discharge	183
Communication	185
Informed Consent	186
Explaining a Procedure	188
Breaking Bad News	189
Consent for a Post-Mortem	191
Drug Adherence	193
Cardio-Pulmonary Resuscitation	195
Adult CPR	196
Paediatric Basic Life Support	198
Procedures	199
Handwash and Scrubbing Up	200
Arterial Blood Gases	203
Measuring Blood Pressure	204
Intravenous Cannulation	206
Venepuncture	207
Male Catheterisation	208
Routine Urinalysis	210
General Topics	211
Confirmation of Death and Death Certification	212
Dermatological Examination	214
Top-Tips: Lymph Node Examination	216
Breast history	217

Breast Examination	219
Preoperative Assessment	222
Examination of an Ulcer	224
Examination of a lump	226
Top-Tips: Looking at fracture X-Rays	228
Top-Tips: Assessment of the acutely ill patient	233
Psychiatry	248
General Psychiatric History and Mental State Assessment	249
Depression History	252
Schizophrenia Assessment	254
Deliberate Self Harm and Suicide Assessment	256
Eyes and Fundoscopy	259
Examination of the Eyes	260
Fundoscopy	263
Ear, Nose and Throat	265
Examination of the Ears	266
Examination of the Nose and Sinuses	267
Examination of the Mouth	268
Gynaecology and Obstetrics	270
General Gynaecological History	271
Obstetric History	274
Bimanual and Smear	277
Top-Tips: Antenatal Obstetrics Examination	280
Paediatrics	282
Neonatal examination	283
Paediatric history	287
References and suggested reading	290

Acknowledgements

The following are experts in their own fields of medicine and have read and amended the contents of this training manual. Their contribution is gratefully acknowledged.

Mr Roger Ackroyd
Consultant Surgeon, Sheffield Teaching Hospitals.
Dr John West
Consultant Cardiologist, Sheffield Teaching Hospitals.
Dr Rod Lawson
Consultant Respiratory Physician, Sheffield Teaching Hospitals.
Dr Andy Gibson
Consultant Neurologist, Sheffield Teaching Hospitals.
Dr Mike Snaith
Senior Lecturer in Rheumatology, Sheffield Teaching Hospitals.
Dr Derek Cullen
Retired Consultant Endocrinologist, Sheffield Teaching Hospitals.
Dr Nusrat Mir
Consultant Psychiatrist, Sheffield Care Trust.
Miss Fiona Kew
Consultant Gynecologist, Jessop Wing, Sheffield Teaching Hospitals.
Mrs Helen Till
Senior Resuscitation Officer, Sheffield Teaching Hospitals.
Mr Senathirajah Muruganinrajah
ENT Surgeon, Sheffield Teaching Hospitals NHS Trust
Mr David Squirrel
Consultant Ophthalmologist, Sheffield Teaching Hospitals NHS Trust
Miss Julia Dicks
SpR in Breast Surgery, Doncaster Royal Infirmary.
Dr Gail Moss
Consultant Paediatrician, Sheffield Childrens Hospital.
Dr David Moore
Consultant Radiologist, Sheffield Teaching Hospitals NHS Trust
Dr Jon Silversides
SpR in Anaesthesia, Royal Victoria Hospital, Belfast.
(Author of 'Assessment of the acutely ill patient')

Background and Design of Objective Structured Clinical Exams
Professor Malcolm Reed

Introduction

Traditionally Medical School clinical final exams included long cases, short cases and viva's. These had advantages in terms of familiarity and to some degree face validity. This meant that the examiners believed that the content of the examination was relevant to the knowledge and skills required of the candidates. However, approximately 20 years ago it was recognised that there were significant weaknesses in these exams. For instance there was a lack of content validity. This means that the exams focused on patients with chronic stable disability who were able to attend for the clinical examinations. This restricted the clinical examination to a very limited assessment of the curriculum, which was not really relevant to the knowledge and skills required to act as a newly qualified doctor. In addition, students felt that these exams were inherently unfair as no two students would undergo the same or even similar examinations in terms of content and range and depth of questioning. More structured examination formats have been developed to address the issues of validity and reliability and the commonest format is the Objective Structured Clinical Examination (OSCE). A major advantage of the OSCE examination is that it permits a wide sampling of the knowledge and skills identified in the curriculum as being relevant to the learning outcomes in undergraduate medical education. Furthermore, all students undergo essentially the same examination, which increases reliability and students feel that these examinations are fair. It is important to recognise that an OSCE exam is not a rigidly defined method of assessment, but represents a structure or framework, which is used to develop a rational assessment of knowledge. OSCE exams are valuable in the direct observation of clinical skills and for the assessment of knowledge, which is not readily assessed in written exams (such as x-rays, etc.). OSCE exams are therefore typically combined with written examinations such as multiple choice, extended matching item and short answer papers. In designing high stakes assessment such as final Medical School examinations it is important to achieve an appropriate balance between the assessment of clinical skills and the underlying knowledge on which clinical practice is based.

How are OSCE exams constructed?

OSCE exams comprise a series of stations in a circuit around which the candidates rotate. At each station the student is required to undertake a clearly defined task. These may include taking a focused history or clinical examination, interpreting an x-ray or performing a practical procedure in simulation. Often a brief period of time is allowed between stations for circulation from one station to the next. This also allows the examiners to complete the mark sheet for each student and for the patient or simulated patient to prepare for the next student. At each station there are clearly defined instructions for the student, which briefly outline the scenario and describe the task that the student is required to undertake. For instance:-

---

Instructions to Candidate

At this station you are required to take a focused history from a patient who presents to the Accident and Emergency Department with severe chest pain.
You have X minutes to complete the task, at which stage the examiners will stop you and ask you to summarise your findings and answer some questions.

It is important that candidates follow the instructions precisely as marks will only be awarded in relation to the task required at that station. For instance at a physical examination station with the following instructions:-

At this station you will meet a patient who presents with a lower abdominal pain. You are required to undertake examination of the abdomen. You have X minutes for this task, at which stage the examiners will stop you and ask you to summarise your findings and ask some questions.

At this station the task clearly relates to performing a physical examination of the abdomen only. Candidates should not take a history or undertake a general examination. However, at all stations candidates will be expected to introduce themselves, outline the purpose of the task, confirm the patient's identity and that they consent to the required task. Candidates should always clean their hands with alcohol-based skin preparation if provided or state to the examiners that this is their normal practice.

Some stations will clarify whether the candidate should describe what they are doing as they proceed with physical examination, but typically a dialogue with the examiner is not required.

For more complex tasks such as information giving stations requiring the candidate to communicate more complex issues with the patient, a preparation station may precede the station where the candidate is examined. Again it is essential that candidates read the information carefully and comply closely with the instructions at the station.

A major advantage of OSCE exams is their flexibility in allowing a wide range of tasks to be assessed. This is greatly extended by the use of simulated patients (actors or volunteers) who are trained to perform a specific role at any station. This increases the number of scenarios, which can be included both in terms of history taking and physical examination. The use of mannequins and simulators extends the range of scenarios even further to include resuscitation and other practical skills. Real patients with clinical signs can also be included in the OSCE examination in the same manner as they were in previous long and short cases, but with the advantage of the interaction being observed and the task structured.

How are OSCE exams put together?

The most important consideration in developing an individual OSCE exam is to make sure that an adequate sample of the syllabus is covered. For a high stakes exam such as a final MBChB exam it is important to ensure that all the relevant aspects of the course are sampled. If it is a lower stakes, end of year or end of module exam then a more focused approach may be appropriate. It is essential that the range and depth of topics to be included in the examination is as transparent as possible in order to avoid students having the sense that there is a hidden syllabus, which has not been formally taught. Therefore, the most effective systems will have assessments at clearly defined points in the course and the body of knowledge and skills to be assessed will be well defined. This applies to both end of year or module exams as well as final examinations.

In order to design an examination, which includes an appropriate sample and spread of content a blue-print is constructed to decide the content of examination. This will help ensure the content validity of the examination and the careful design of individual questions and the inclusion of a suitable number of stations will help ensure the reliability of the exam.

Constructing the Blue-print

This task is usually undertaken several months before the examination. A standard blue-print is developed, which is essentially a matrix of the content, skills and knowledge to be assessed. One axis of the matrix comprises the areas to be assessed (e.g. history taking, physical examination, practical procedures, etc). The other axis of the matrix typically covers the clinical systems in which these skills may be evaluated (e.g. cardiovascular, respiratory, musculoskeletal, etc.). Many schools will also have a defined list of problems, which can be incorporated into this axis of the matrix. Once a standard matrix is developed then the exam can be designed by use of an appropriate sampling process (see Appendix 1). Appropriate scenarios from the problem list can then be defined and OSCE questions either selected from a bank of questions or new questions developed specifically for the examination. This process represents a structured approach to designing the exam ensuring that all the competences are assessed and that all body systems are included in the examination with an appropriate spread of clinical problems. It is important to cross reference the development of the OSCE blueprint with a similar process for developing the written components of the examination to ensure that there is not excessive emphasis in any one area of knowledge or body systems.

It is possible to internally weight the exam to ensure that the more important body systems and clinical problems are adequately assessed. For instance two or three scenarios assessing knowledge in the cardiovascular and respiratory systems may be included whereas only one may be included in less commonly encountered areas such as endocrinology. Generally speaking greater reliability is achieved by having more scenarios in an examination rather than by having longer stations or more than one examiner at any given station. Individual examinations vary but the length of stations may be anywhere between five and fifteen minutes with many schools now moving towards ten minutes or longer stations. A minimum examining time would be one and a half to two hours with some schools running considerably longer assessments. There are a number of variations of OSCE examinations with various titles but the essential components described above are commonly regarded as good practice in terms of designing these assessments.

Marking OSCE Stations

There are broadly two types of marking systems utilised and increasingly these are combined in OSCE examinations. The first approach is to have a list of key points or items that the students should perform (itemised mark sheets). These are common in undergraduate assessments particularly in the early clinical years. Typical examples of these are included in the chapters of this textbook. Key points may include a series of individual actions in performing a physical examination or points to be covered in taking a history. Itemised mark sheets also lend themselves particularly well to the assessment of practical procedures.

Increasingly marking schemes also incorporate more global overall judgements about the performance of a student at an individual station. In addition to scoring individual items at the station the examiner also awards a mark for the overall approach to the task. In communication skill stations it is common for the real or simulated patient to contribute to the mark achieved by the student. When experienced examiners are marking OSCE exams the use of global ratings is an alternative approach. This is because the use of mark sheets with multiple items to be ticked off by the examiners can distract them from observing the candidate's performance and restrict them from making a judgement on how well the candidate performs the tasks as well as how comprehensive they are in terms of covering the expected knowledge or skills at the station. An example of a hybrid mark sheet commonly used in undergraduate assessments is included as Appendix 2.

How to Approach a Final Year OSCE Exam

Remember that the clinical examination predominantly assesses clinical skills and therefore the appropriate setting to prepare for this examination is in the ward, outpatients or general practice. The skills required are obtained and refined through practice rather than revising in the library. Ensure that you have observed experienced doctors as much as possible and have practiced your clinical skills and relevant clinical skills in simulation extensively before the examination. An experienced examiner can tell in a very short period of time if a candidate is performing a task for the first time!

Read all the materials provided for you by the school carefully in preparation for the examination. Most schools will provide detailed information in the course handbook about how the exams are structured.

Typically there are no 'killer' stations or key individual points within a station which must be completed in order to pass.

It is likely that a student's will vary at different stations as the exam is designed to assess both the breadth and depth of your knowledge. If you feel a station has not gone well then try not to let this put you off for the rest of the examination. The examiners do not confer with each other from one station to the next and a poor performance at one station is not carried over for the rest of the exam. Follow the individual instructions at each station very carefully. The marks are only awarded for the task that is required. If anything is unclear ask the examiners for clarification but do not expect them to 'coax' the correct answer from you. Remember this is not primarily a viva or dialogue between you and the examiner. The focus is on your interactions with patients.

Always remember to demonstrate professional attitudes and behaviours in your interactions with patients and examiners. These can represent a significant contribution to the mark scheme.

Remember that the content and tables in this text are designed to act as an aide memoir. You do not necessarily need to "rattle through" all the questions included in each section of this book but should be careful to focus your questioning or examination closely to the task required at each station. Select carefully from the lists those points which are relevant to the scenario at any given station. You are likely to be asked to present and summarize what you have found at the end – this is to assess whether you can synthesize and communicate complex information. Remember to provide a concise summary rather than recite the whole history. The examiner may then ask about your differential diagnosis and management plan for each patient encountered.

Good Luck!

Malcolm Reed

Sampling Process (Theoretical)

Competence Categories	CVS	RS	CNS	Mental Health	MSS	GI	Endo/ Repro	Haem/ Onc/Inf	Renal/ Metab	Eyes/ENT	Skin/ Misc
History Taking	Chest Pain						Vaginal Discharge				
Physical Exam		Shortness of Breath						Enlarged Spleen			
Tests and Procedures			Weakness						Haematuria		
Data Interpretation				Sleep Disturbance						Visual Disturbance	
Management					Trauma						Hair Loss
Communication and Patient Education						Rectal Bleeding					

EXAMINERS NAME ....   **STUDENT NAME**

(BLOCK CAPITALS)

AFFIX LABEL HERE

STATION No.

PHYSICAL EXAMINATION

MARK SHEET

Greet the student and give him/her the written instructions.

REMEMBER TO ASK THE STUDENT FOR THEIR IDENTITY LABEL AND AFFIX IT TO THE TOP OF THE MARK SHEET.

Please circle the appropriate mark for each criterion. The standard expected is that of a new PRHO.

Example of task	Performed competently	Performed but not fully competent	Not performed or incompetent
Initial approach to the patient (introduces him-herself, explains what he/she will be doing)	2	1	0

Overall approach to task	4	3	2	1	0

Overall Rating:

Clear Fail	Borderline	Clear Pass

Examiners Signature...

Tips and advice

- Read the written instructions or case scenarios carefully. Always stick to them and perform the task as exactly asked in the statement.
- If uncertain of the instructions check with the examiner. You *must* clarify any uncertainties before you start your task.
- Remember your professional interaction with the patient. Examiners always look for it. Introduce yourself and refer to the patient by name, this is stressed in each examination section of this book. Don't rush. In communication stations listen to the patients first. They have scripted instructions. Start with an open question and listen, they will be cueing you the information. Ask about concerns. If asked to give an explanation always find out what the patient understands first. Never dive straight in.
- Be considerate and gentle when examining patients. Examiners get very upset if patients are not treated with respect. There is often an overall mark (global rating) as well as a checklist where they may mark you down for this.
- Study equipment carefully. As you start a practical skills procedure check the equipment. If you see a sharps box or yellow disposal bag you can be sure there will be a mark for using it.
- Avoid watching the examiners ticking boxes. This can be very misleading. Practising the tables in this book with your friends will take a lot of this scare away.
- Timing. If you are given warning bells - for example, one more minute, use the time to summarise and conclude the OSCE station. There are often marks for this.
- It is normal to be anxious but take a deep breath and stay calm. Focus on the task ahead. Use rest stations to think forwards not backwards.

Adapted from sBMJ;2000 Oct:361-362 with permission from the BMJ Publishing Group

How to use this book

1.   The first and foremost advice is to try and familiarise yourself with the tables and practice them frequently enough that they can be repeated automatically from memory.

2.   We suggest that you should organise yourselves in groups of 3 students each. One student can be the examiner, one students the candidate and the third student can be the mock patient. You can then rotate the examiner, candidate and patients so that everyone gets a chance to practice their clinical skills.

3.   Create your own clinical scenario based on the common symptoms we have covered in this book. For example:

"A 45 year old man presents to the Accident and Emergency Department with shortness of breath. Please take a history from this patient"

or

"Examine this patient's respiratory system".

4.   The "student" should be given the clinical scenario and proceed to take a history or conduct an examination as required. The "examiner" should have this book and score the performance of the "candidate" against the table provided.

5.   At the end of a five-minute station, a total mark can be calculated and feedback can be given to the "candidate" regarding any points in the history or examination that they have missed.

The importance of repeated practice cannot be stressed enough because that is the only way you will reduce omissions from your examination.

We have included explanatory remarks to help you understand the importance of various points in the history or steps in the clinical examination.

Abbreviations Used

ACE	Angiotensin converting enzyme
ACTH	Adrenocorticotrophic hormone
ADH	Anti-diuretic hormone
CABG	Coronary artery bypass graft
CN	Cranial nerve
COPD	Chronic obstructive pulmonary disease
DIP	Distal interphalangeal joint
DM	Diabetes mellitus
DOB	Date of birth
DVT	Deep venous thrombosis
GI	Gastrointestinal
GOR	Gastro-oesophageal reflux
HBV	Hepatitis B virus
HCV	Hepatitis C virus
INR	International normalised ratio
IVC	Inferior vena cava
JVP	Jugular venous pressure
LA	Left atrium
LBBB	Left bundle branch block
LMN	Lower motor neurone
LV	Left ventricle
MCP	Metacarpophalangeal joint
MI	Myocardial infarction
MND	Motor neurone disease
MS	Multiple sclerosis
NSAIDs	Non-steroidal anti-inflammatory drugs
pCO_2	Partial pressure of carbon dioxide
PCOS	Polycystic ovary syndrome
PE	Pulmonary embolus
PIP	Proximal interphalangeal joint
PND	Paroxysmal nocturnal dyspnoea
RA	Right atrium
RBBB	Right bundle branch block
RV	Right ventricle
SVC	Superior vena cava
TIA	Transient ischaemic attack
UMN	Upper motor neurone
UTI	Urinary tract infection
VSD	Ventricular septal defect

The Gastrointestinal System

General Gastrointestinal System History

		Not attempted	Attempted inadequate	Attempted adequate
1	Approaches the patient politely and introduces him/herself.	0	1	2
2	Asks the patient's name, DOB and occupation.	0	1	2
3	Asks about history of abdominal pain.	0	1	2
4	Asks about history of nausea, vomiting or haematemesis.	0	1	2
5	Asks about history of dysphagia.	0	1	2
6	Asks about history of heartburn or dyspepsia.	0	1	2
7	Asks about history of diarrhoea, constipation of a recent change in bowel habit.	0	1	2
8	Asks about history of bleeding per rectum.	0	1	2
9	Asks about weight loss and loss of appetite.	0	1	2
10	Asks about history of jaundice, yellow sclerae, pale stools and dark urine.	0	1	2
11	Asks about recurring mouth ulcers	0	1	2
12	Asks about past or current medical conditions and previous abdominal surgery.	0	1	2
13	Asks about family history of bowel cancer or other bowel disorders.	0	1	2
14	Asks about home circumstances.	0	1	2
15	Asks about smoking and alcohol consumption.	0	1	2
16	Asks about past and current medications and any allergies to medication.	0	1	2

1. It is polite and professional to introduce yourself.

2. Name: to establish rapport and identify the patient.
   Age/DOB: certain diseases affect certain age groups, e.g. colon cancer is rare in the young. The date of birth should be recorded to identify the patient.
   Occupation: this can tell you a lot about the patient's background and can have significant effects on the management of their condition. It may also be relevant to the aetiology of the condition e.g. hepatitis in health care workers.

3. See specific history for abdominal pain.

4. See specific history for nausea or vomiting.

5. See specific history for dysphagia.

6. See specific history for dyspepsia.

7. See specific history for change in bowel habit.

8. See specific history for bleeding per rectum.

9. The presence of both anorexia and weight loss should alert you to the possibility of a malignancy (but may also occur with depression and other diseases). Weight loss with increased appetite suggests malabsorption or a hypermetabolic state.

10. See specific history for jaundice.

11. Mouth ulcers especially if recurring, can be a symptom of Crohn's disease or ulcerative colitis

12. Medical conditions (e.g. atrial fibrillation) and previous surgery may provide important clues to the diagnosis.
Enquire about conditions such as inflammatory bowel disease, which run a chronic course punctuated by exacerbations.
A past history of relapsing epigastric pain in a patient presenting with severe abdominal pain may indicate that a long-standing peptic ulcer has perforated. Abdominal surgical procedures can result in adhesions which may cause intestinal obstruction. Occasionally, damage to the bile duct at cholecystectomy might cause a biliary stricture resulting in jaundice.
It is important to consider other systems as well e.g. a goitre with retrosternal extension can be a cause of dysphagia. Many endocrine and metabolic disturbances are associated with a change in bowel habit.

13. The hereditary condition of familial adenomatous polyposis predisposes to colorectal cancer.

14. The diagnosis of a chronic illness can have serious psychological effects and a patient's home circumstances can affect their ability to cope.
In the case of infectious conditions, it is necessary to enquire about other household members.

15. Alcohol can cause a wide spectrum of liver disease from fatty change to hepatitis and cirrhosis. It can also cause vomiting, chronic pancreatitis, ulcers and upper GI bleeding.
Cigarette smoking is associated with an increased risk of gastric and oesophageal cancer. Smoking also worsens GOR. Patients with Crohn's disease are more likely to be tobacco smokers.

16. NSAIDs can induce GI bleeding.
Codeine preparations and some antidepressants can cause constipation.
The liver can be damaged by many drugs including phenytoin, tetracyclines and amiodarone. An overdose of paracetamol can cause acute liver cell necrosis.
Cholestasis may result from hypersensivity reactions to chlorpromazine, sulponamides, sulphonylureas, rifampacin, nitrofurantoin or the combined contraceptive pill.
Anticholinergics, calcium channel blockers, theophylline and nitrates are known to increase GOR.
A large number of drugs can induce vomiting including opiates, dopamine agonists and cytotoxics.

Presenting Complaint - Abdominal Pain

		Not attempted	Attempted inadequate	Attempted adequate
1	Asks the patient to point to where the pain is worst.	0	1	2
2	Asks the patient whether the pain radiates anywhere.	0	1	2
3	Asks the patient to describe the character of the pain.	0	1	2
4	Asks the patient about the onset and duration of the pain.	0	1	2
5	Asks the patient to rate the severity of the pain.	0	1	2
6	Asks whether the pain is intermittent or constant.	0	1	2
7	Asks whether there is anything that makes the pain better or worse e.g. movement or coughing.	0	1	2
8	Asks whether there is any relationship to food, particularly fatty food.	0	1	2
9	Asks if there is any associated nausea, vomiting or abdominal distension.	0	1	2
10	Asks if there has been any change in bowel habit, when the patient last had their bowels open and whether the motion was normal for them.	0	1	2
11	Asks whether the patient feels systemically unwell, has a fever or suffers from night sweats.	0	1	2
12	Asks whether they have eaten anything unusual or undercooked in the past few days and if any other family member has had similar symptoms.	0	1	2
13	Asks whether they have noticed any weight loss.	0	1	2
14	Asks whether there is any associated jaundice with the pain. Asks about pale stools, dark urine and yellow sclerae.	0	1	2
15	Asks about urinary symptoms, particularly haematuria and dysuria.	0	1	2
16	If the patient is female, asks when her last menstrual period was and whether there is any chance that she could be pregnant.	0	1	2
17	Asks about drug treatment and specifically if the patient takes NSAIDs regularly.	0	1	2
18	Asks about previous abdominal surgery and history of groin lumps.	0	1	2

1. The site of the pain gives a clue as to the underlying organ involved.

2. Pain radiating to the back is characteristic of pancreatic disease, a perforated peptic ulcer or a ruptured abdominal aneurysm.
   The pain of oesophageal reflux radiates up to the neck whilst that of renal colic radiates from loin to groin.
   The sensation of diaphragmatic irritation is referred to the shoulder tip.

3. Colicky pain results from obstruction of a hollow viscus (bowel, ureter).
   A dull or burning pain may be caused by peptic ulceration.

4. Determine whether the pain is acute, chronic or acute on chronic.
   An acute episode on a background of chronic dull pain might indicate recurrent pancreatitis or perforation of a peptic ulcer.
   If a patient is presenting with chronic pain, try to determine what it is that has prompted them to seek help now.

5. Ask the patient to rate their pain as mild, moderate or severe.

6. Peptic ulcer disease produces episodic pain whereas pancreatic pain is usually steady. Biliary pain can last for hours.

7. Patients attempt to relieve colicky pain by rolling around vigorously whereas peritonitis is aggravated by movement or coughing.
   Antacids or vomiting may relieve pain due to peptic ulcers or gastro-oesophageal reflux.
   Defecation or passage of flatus may relieve the pain of irritable bowel disease.
   Pancreatic pain is characteristically relieved by sitting and leaning forwards.

8. Eating may precipitate pain from a gastric ulcer but relieve that due to a duodenal ulcer. Fatty foods are thought to precipitate gallbladder pain.

9. Vomiting can be a feature of the pathological process itself, as in intestinal obstruction, or can be related to pain, particularly if it is severe as in biliary or renal colic.

10. A chronic erratic disturbance of defecation associated with abdominal pain and bloating is characteristic of irritable bowel syndrome.
    Recent constipation or diarrhoea associated with colicky pain may point to large bowel malignancy or stricture formation. Often there will be blood or mucous passed with the stool.
    Rectal malignancies typically cause increased frequency of defecation and a sense of incomplete evacuation, known as tenesmus.
    Inflammatory bowel disease causes diarrhoea in association with abdominal pain.

11. Pyrexia and night sweats in particular point to an infective cause.

12. Find out whether the patient has been abroad recently and eaten anything unusual or whether they have eaten anything that they felt was a possible cause of gastrointestinal upset. Vomiting and diarrhoea together, especially in more than one member of a family, points to infective gastroenteritis.

13. Weight loss may suggest an underlying malignancy.

14. Jaundice associated with biliary pain suggests gallstones.

15. Urinary symptoms associated with pain typical of renal colic suggest stones in the urinary tract.

16. Causes of abdominal pain in early pregnancy include threatened abortion and ruptured ectopic pregnancy, which can occur before the patient realises that they are pregnant.

17. NSAIDs exacerbate peptic ulceration.

18. Abdominal surgery can result in adhesions leading to obstruction and pain. Irreducible herniae are a common cause of small bowel obstruction.

Medical Causes of Abdominal Pain

"ABDOMENAL PANE" [abdominal pain]:
Acute rheumatic fever
Blood [purpura, a/c hemolytic crisis]
DKA
c**O**llagen vascular disease
Migraine [abdominal migraine]
Epilepsy [abdominal epilepsy]
Nephron [uremia]
Abdominal angina
Lead
Porphyria
Arsenic
NSAID's
Enteric fever

Presenting Complaint - Dysphagia

		Not attempted	Attempted inadequate	Attempted adequate
1	Asks the patient how long they have had difficulty swallowing and if it is getting worse or staying the same.	0	1	2
2	Asks if swallowing is painful.	0	1	2
3	Asks the patient where food appears to stick.	0	1	2
4	Asks whether they have difficulty with liquids as well as solids.	0	1	2
5	Asks whether the difficulty eases after the first few swallows.	0	1	2
6	Asks whether fluid ever regurgitates into the throat or causes the patient to choke.	0	1	2
7	Asks about weight loss and loss of appetite.	0	1	2
8	Asks about history of heartburn.	0	1	2
9	Asks whether they have noticed any lumps in their neck.	0	1	2
10	Asks whether they have a cough, feel short of breath or have noticed their voice becoming hoarse.	0	1	2
11	Asks whether the patient smokes and how much alcohol they drink.			
12	Asks whether the patient has been taking antibiotics.			

1. Progressive difficulty in swallowing suggests a carcinoma or stricture formation whilst intermittent difficulty suggests a motility disorder such as achalasia. Rapid progression of dysphagia is a sinister sign.

2. Odynophagia occurs with infection of the oesophagus (eg. with candida or herpes simplex) or with ulceration of the oesophagus.

3. A sensation of food sticking in the oesophagus may indicate a blockage. Obstruction high in the oesophagus may be felt anywhere in the upper retrosternal area whereas obstruction lower in the oesophagus will usually be felt in the lower retrosternal or epigastric area.

4. Intermittent difficulty in swallowing both liquids and solids points to achalasia or diffuse oesophageal spasm.
   Dysphagia which is initially for solids only but then progresses to liquids is more likely to be due to a stricture or carcinoma.

5. If the dysphagia eases after the first few swallows, it is probably due to oesophageal spasm.

6. Fluid regurgitating into the throat or nose suggests that the cause of the dysphagia is in the pharynx eg. neurological disease such as MND. Severe GOR may also cause regurgitation or waterbrash.

7. Associated weight loss suggests carcinoma of the oesophagus or gastric cardia (if it is not simply due to decreased intake).

8. GOR predisposes to both stricture formation and the development of oesophageal carcinoma.

9. A retrosternal goitre can be a cause of dysphagia.
   Virchow's nodes in the supraclavicular area might indicate a carcinoma of the oesophagus or stomach (Troisier's sign)

10. Bronchial carcinoma can be a cause of dysphagia and also causes cough, dyspnoea and hoarseness (if it affects the recurrent laryngeal nerve).

11. Smoking and excessive alcohol intake are risk factors for oesophageal carcinoma.

12. Tetracyclines can cause oesophageal irritation and dysphagia.

Presenting Complaint – Dyspepsia

		Not attempted	Attempted inadequate	Attempted adequate
1	Asks the patient to describe the sensation of indigestion that they feel.	0	1	2
2	Asks whether the patient notices it particularly after certain food or drinks.	0	1	2
3	Asks if bending, stooping or lying down aggravates the symptoms.	0	1	2
4	Asks the patient whether there is anything that relieves the indigestion or heartburn.	0	1	2
5	Asks whether they ever get a sour or bitter tasting fluid coming up into their mouth.	0	1	2
6	Asks if they have been vomiting.	0	1	2
7	Asks if they have noticed any weight loss.	0	1	2
8	Asks if they have vomited blood or noticed any blood in their stool or whether they pass black tarry stool.	0	1	2
9	Asks whether the patient has noticed feeling unusually full after small amounts of food.	0	1	2
10	Asks whether the patient feels bloated especially after meals	0	1	2

1. Indigestion is a term often used to describe any symptom (nausea, heartburn, bloating etc.) occurring after food or drink. It is important to clarify the exact nature of the patient's complaint.

2. Reflux symptoms are aggravated by alcohol, chocolate, caffeine and fatty meals.

3. These postural changes are also known to aggravate the symptoms of GOR.

4. Antacids transiently relieve the pain caused GOR.

5. Acid regurgitation is a symptom that strongly suggests that GOR is occurring.

6. Indigestion can be a symptom of gastric cancer, which if in the pyloric area, can also lead to vomiting.

7. Weight loss may suggest a malignancy.

8. Haematemesis and malaena can result from erosion of the mucosa over a gastric tumour or be due to a bleeding peptic ulcer.

9. Early satiety can result from a gastric cancer.

10. Bloating can be a symptom of irritable bowel.

Presenting Complaint - Vomiting

		Not attempted	Attempted inadequate	Attempted adequate
1	Asks the patient how often they have been vomiting.	0	1	2
2	Asks whether the vomiting was of sudden onset or if it has been longstanding.	0	1	2
3	Asks the patient whether they vomit at any particular time of day and if anything brings the episodes on.	0	1	2
4	Asks whether the vomiting is related to abdominal pain and if so, whether the vomiting relieves the pain.	0	1	2
5	Asks how much the patient brings up and if the vomiting is projectile.	0	1	2
6	Asks what colour the vomit is.	0	1	2
7	Asks whether the vomit ever looks like coffee grounds or is blood stained.	0	1	2
8	Asks whether the vomit contains residues of food taken the day before.	0	1	2
9	Asks whether the patient feels systemically unwell or has any other symptoms.	0	1	2
10	Asks whether they have eaten anything unusual in the past few days and if any other family member has similar symptoms.			
11	Asks whether there has been any recent change in bowel habit.	0	1	2
12	Asks about appetite and whether there is early satiety.	0	1	2
13	If the patient is female, asks if there is any possibility that they could be pregnant.			
14	Asks specifically about alcohol consumption.	0	1	2

1. This helps to determine the severity and the immediate management. A patient who has been vomiting very frequently will be dehydrated and metabolically deranged and need urgent attention.

2. Acute symptoms are most likely to be caused by infections (including food poisoning), or small bowel obstruction.
   Vomiting can also be associated with pregnancy, drugs, peptic ulcer disease with gastric outlet obstruction, hepatobiliary disease, alcoholism, raised intracranial pressure and psychogenic disorders.

3. Early morning vomiting is characteristic of pregnancy, alcoholism and raised intracranial pressure.
   Vomiting delayed by more than one hour after a meal is characteristic of

gastric outlet obstruction or gastroparesis.

4. Pancreatitis, small bowel obstruction and biliary disease can cause both abdominal pain and vomiting.
    Nausea and vomiting without pain may be non-gastrointestinal in origin.

5. Large volumes of vomit suggest intestinal obstruction. Projectile vomiting is typical of gastric outlet obstruction.

6. Bilious vomit (green) suggests small bowel obstruction.
    Red / brown vomit may be stained by blood.
    Faeculent vomit is a late sign of distal small bowel or large bowel obstruction.

7. Blood in the vomit is usually a sign of ulceration of the upper GI tract. It may have the appearance of coffee grounds.

8. Old food in the vomit suggests gastric outlet obstruction.

9. Systemic upset, such as pyrexia and night sweats, points to an infectious cause for the vomiting.
    Morning headaches in conjunction with vomiting are symptoms of raised intracranial pressure.

10. Symptoms in close contacts suggest an infectious cause is likely. It is important to identify the likely source of any suspected food poisoning.

11. Acute diarrhoea associated with vomiting suggests an infective cause.
    Constipation associated with vomiting suggests intestinal obstruction.

12. Asking about appetite may be helpful in determining whether there is any eating disorder such as bulimia nervosa.
    Early satiety may be due to a gastric neoplasm.

13. Vomiting is a common symptom of early pregnancy.

14. Vomiting is a feature of both acute alcohol intoxication and chronic excess.

Causes of vomiting

VOMITING
Vestibular disturbance/ **V**agal (reflex pain)
Opiates
Migrane/ **M**etabolic (DKA, gastroparesis, hypercalcemia)
Infections
Toxicity (cytotoxic, digitalis toxicity)
Increased ICP, **I**ngested alcohol
Neurogenic, psychogenic
Gestation

Presenting Complaint - Jaundice

		Not attempted	Attempted inadequate	Attempted adequate
1	Asks when the patient first noticed yellowing of their eyes or skin and if it is progressive or fluctuating.	0	1	2
2	Asks the patient whether there has been a change in colour of their stool or urine and if so, what colour they are.	0	1	2
3	Asks if the patient has any abdominal pain.	0	1	2
4	Asks if the patient has noticed any weight loss.	0	1	2
5	Asks whether their skin itches.	0	1	2
6	Asks whether they have vomited at all.	0	1	2
7	Asks the patient whether they bruise or bleed easily.	0	1	2
8	Asks the patient how much alcohol they drink.	0	1	2
9	Asks whether the patient has travelled abroad recently and if so, where to.	0	1	2
10	Asks if they have had any recent surgery.	0	1	2
11	Asks if the patient has ever had a blood transfusion.	0	1	2
12	Tactfully asks the patient whether they have abused drugs and whether they are homosexual.	0	1	2

1. A history of progressive jaundice, particularly if associated with weight loss, is suggestive of a malignancy or chronic liver disease.
   A short history, particularly with a prodromal illness, may suggest hepatitis or gallstones.
   Fluctuating jaundice is usually associated with bile duct stones.

2. Pale stools and dark urine occur in obstructive jaundice because less bilirubin reaches the intestine and there is increased renal excretion.

3. Abdominal pain in association with jaundice is suggestive of gallstones.

4. Weight loss associated with the jaundice suggests malignancy or chronic liver disease.

5. Cholestatic liver disease can cause pruritis, which tends to be worse over the extremities.

6. Acute hepatobiliary disease can cause both jaundice and vomiting. Advanced carcinoma of the head of the pancreas can cause duodenal obstruction leading to vomiting.

7. Obstructive jaundice results in a shortage of bile salts (which emulsify fat) in the intestine and therefore reduces the absorption of vitamin K (which is a fat-soluble

vitamin). This decreases the production of clotting factors II, VII, IX and X and the patient may therefore bleed and bruise easily.

8. Alcoholic liver disease can lead to jaundice.

9. The incidence of viral hepatitis varies geographically. Africa and parts of Asia have the highest carrier rates of hepatitis B and C. Hepatitis A occurs in epidemics worldwide.

10. Iatrogenic injury to the biliary tract can result in jaundice.

11. HBV and HCV can be transmitted by blood and blood products.

12. Male homosexuality increases the risk of HBV infection whereas intravenous drug abuse increases the chance of HBV and HCV infection.

Presenting Complaint - Diarrhoea

		Not attempted	Attempted inadequate	Attempted adequate
1	Asks the patient how often they pass motions currently and what the patient feels is normal for them.	0	1	2
2	Asks when the patient's bowel habit first changed.	0	1	2
3	Asks if there is any relationship between the diarrhoea and meals.	0	1	2
4	Asks what colour the motions are.	0	1	2
5	Asks whether the stool is formed or watery.	0	1	2
6	Asks whether the patient has ever passed any blood or mucus.	0	1	2
7	Asks whether the stools float in the lavatory or are difficult to flush away or smell excessively foul.	0	1	2
8	Asks whether the patient has any abdominal pain and if so, if passing of motions or flatus relieves it.	0	1	2
9	Asks about weight loss and loss of appetite.	0	1	2
10	Asks whether the patient has also been vomiting.	0	1	2
11	Asks about recent travel and any change in diet.	0	1	2
12	Asks if the patient suffers from bloating or abdominal distension.	0	1	2
13	Asks about symptoms of thyroid disease.	0	1	2
14	Asks whether the patient has ever been incontinent.	0	1	2
15	Asks if the patient is on any medications.	0	1	2
16	Asks whether the patient has been feeling particularly tired or short of breath recently.	0	1	2
17	Asks if there is a family history of bowel cancer or inflammatory bowel disease.			

1. It is always important to find out what is normal in terms of bowel habit for each individual patient. True diarrhoea is defined as the passing of increased amounts of loose stool.

2. Acute diarrhoea is likely to be infective in nature.
   Chronic diarrhoea can be related to irritable bowel or a metabolic or endocrine disturbance.

3. Secretory diarrhoea (caused by infections or carcinoid syndrome) persists when the patient fasts.
   Osmotic diarrhoea (caused by lactose intolerance, magnesium antacids or after gastric surgery) is characterised by large volume stools related to the ingestion of food.

4. Steatorrhoea consists of pale, foul smelling stools.
   Stool containing blood can vary from bright red to black.

5. Secretory and osmotic diarrhoea are both characterised by loose, watery stools. Some patients may pass small amounts of formed stool several times a day because of increased desire to defaecate but this is not true diarrhoea.

6. Mucus in the stool may be due to a rectal ulcer, fistula or villous adenoma or occur as part of irritable bowel syndrome.
   Blood present in the stool can be arising from anywhere in the GI tract.

7. Offensive smelling stools, which float in the toilet bowl, are typical of steatorrhoea which is a feature of malabsorption syndromes.

8. The pain of diverticulitis or irritable bowel may be temporarily relieved by the passage of flatus or by defecation.

9. Weight loss and loss of appetite in this context are suggestive of a malignancy.

10. Vomiting associated with diarrhoea suggests an infective cause.

11. Travel and diet are important clues as to the likely organism involved in infective gastroenteritis.

12. Intermittent abdominal distension associated with diarrhoea is characteristic of irritable bowel syndrome.

13. Diarrhoea is a symptom of thyrotoxicosis.

14. Faecal incontinence can be caused a large number of conditions including faceal impaction with overflow diarrhoea, anorectal disease (eg. prolapse, rectal carcinoma), post-childbirth pelvic floor trauma, neurological disorders (eg. trauma at level of S2 - S4, MS), senile dementia or diabetes mellitus with autonomic involvement.

15. Many drugs, including many types of antibiotic, can cause diarrhoea.

16. Colorectal cancer can lead to anaemia.

17. Both of these conditions have hereditary links.

Presenting Complaint - Constipation

		Not attempted	Attempted inadequate	Attempted adequate
1	Asks the patient how often they pass motions currently and what the patient feels is normal for them.	0	1	2
2	Asks when the patient's bowel habit first changed.	0	1	2
3	Asks what colour the motions are.	0	1	2
4	Asks whether the patient has ever passed any blood or mucus.	0	1	2
5	Asks whether the patient has any abdominal pain and if so, if passing of motions or flatus relieves it.	0	1	2
6	Asks whether the patient has pain on defecation.	0	1	2
7	Asks whether the patient has to strain or gets a feeling of incomplete emptying of the rectum.	0	1	2
8	Asks about weight loss and loss of appetite.	0	1	2
9	Asks whether the patient has ever been incontinent.	0	1	2
10	Asks whether the patient has been vomiting.	0	1	2
11	Asks if the patient is on any medications.	0	1	2
12	Asks whether the patient has been feeling particularly tired or short of breath recently.	0	1	2
13	Asks whether there is any family history of bowel cancer or inflammatory bowel disease.	0	1	2

1. Constipation can refer to the infrequent passage of stool or the difficult passage of hard stools, irrespective of the frequency.

2. Chronic constipation may arise because of habitual neglect of the impulse to defaecate or from drugs, metabolic or endocrine disease or abnormal colonic motility. Recent onset constipation may be due to development of a malignancy.

3. Steatorrhoea consists of pale, foul smelling stools.
   Stool containing blood can vary from bright red to black.

4. Mucus in the stool may be due to a rectal ulcer, fistula or villous adenoma or occur as part of irritable bowel syndrome.
   There are a large number of causes of blood in the stool.

5. The pain of colonic diverticular disease or irritable bowel may be temporarily relieved by the passage of flatus or by defecation.

6. Pain on defecation may indicate an anal lesion such as a fissure.

7. Disorders of the pelvic floor muscles or nerves or anorectal disease may lead to straining or even the need to self-digitate. A feeling of incomplete emptying is a symptom of rectal cancer.

8. Weight loss and loss of appetite are suggestive of a malignancy.

9. Faecal incontinence can be caused a large number of conditions including faceal impaction with overflow diarrhoea, anorectal disease (eg. prolapse, rectal carcinoma), post-childbirth pelvic floor trauma, neurological disorders (eg. trauma at level of S2 - S4, MS), senile dementia or diabetes mellitus with autonomic involvement.

10. Vomiting associated with constipation suggests intestinal obstruction.

11. Opiates cause constipation.

12. Colorectal cancer can lead to anaemia.

13. Both of these conditions have hereditary links.

Presenting Complaint - Rectal Bleeding

		Not attempted	Attempted inadequate	Attempted adequate
1	Asks the patient when they first noticed blood in their stool.	0	1	2
2	Asks what colour the blood was.	0	1	2
3	Asks whether the blood was mixed in with the stool, on the outside of the stool, in the toilet bowl or on the toilet paper.	0	1	2
4	Asks whether there has been any associated change in bowel habit.	0	1	2
5	Asks whether the patient has passed any mucous or slime with the blood.	0	1	2
6	Asks whether there is any associated abdominal pain.	0	1	2
7	Asks whether defecation is painful.	0	1	2
8	Asks whether the patient has a history of haemorrhoids.	0	1	2
9	Asks about weight loss and loss of appetite.	0	1	2
10	Asks whether they ever notice a feeling of 'something coming down' or a 'dragging sensation'.	0	1	2
11	Asks whether the patient is passing urine normally.	0	1	2
12	Asks specifically whether they are on warfarin.			
13	Asks whether the patient has been feeling particularly tired or short of breath recently.			
14	Asks whether there is any family history of bowel cancer or inflammatory bowel disease.			

1. It is important to determine whether there has been an acute bleed or whether there has been chronic blood loss into the stool.

2. Bright red blood indicates that it is coming from the anus or rectum whereas darker blood indicates that it is originating from higher up the GI tract.

3. Anorectal disease typically leads to blood on the outside of the stool or noticed on the toilet paper. Lesions higher up in the GI tract lead to the blood being mixed in with the stool.

4. An associated change in bowel habit raises the possibility of a malignancy.

5. Mucus being passed with bloody stool suggests that the underlying lesion may be a rectal ulcer or proctitis.

6. Causes of rectal bleeding that also cause abdominal pain include colorectal carcinoma, inflammatory bowel disease, intussusception, massive upper GI haemorrhage or diverticular disease.

7. Painful defecation suggests that there may be an anal fissure.

8. Haemorrhoids cause bleeding which is noticed as blood on the toilet paper.

9. Weight loss and loss of appetite in conjunction with rectal bleeding suggests that there may be a malignancy.

10. These are phrases often used to describe the sensation cause by a prolapse. Rectal prolapse will cause bleeding if the overlying mucosa becomes eroded.

11. If a patient also has urinary problems then there could be a colonic tumour pressing on the bladder or the underlying problem could be prostatic carcinoma invading the rectal wall.

12. If a patient's INR is too high, they will bleed more readily from any potential bleeding site.

13. Chronic occult rectal bleeding may lead to anaemia.

14. Both of these conditions have hereditary links.

Macrocytic Anaemia

ABCDEF:
Alcohol + liver disease
B12 deficiency
Compensatory reticulocytosis (blood loss and haemolysis)
Drug (cytotoxic and AZT)/ **D**ysplasia (marrow problems)
Endocrine (hypothyroidism)
Folate deficiency/ **F**etus (pregnancy)

Examination Of The Gastrointestinal System

		Not attempted	Attempted inadequate	Attempted adequate
1	Approaches the patient politely and introduces him/herself. Washes hands. Positions patient on bed and exposes the patient from nipples to knees after obtaining their permission. Asks for a chaperone.	0	1	2
2	Performs a general inspection from the end of the bed.	0	1	2
3	Feels the radial pulse, commenting on rate and regularity.	0	1	2
4	Inspects the nails and hands commenting on clubbing, koilonychia, leuconychia, palmar erythema and Dupytrens contracture.	0	1	2
5	Tests for hepatic flap in the hands and looks at the arms for bruising and scratch marks.	0	1	2
6	Looks at the eyes commenting on jaundice, pallor or Kayser-Fleischer rings.	0	1	2
7	Looks with a torch around and inside the mouth commenting on angular stomatitis, circumoral pigmentation, telangiectasiae, ulcers and glossitis. Also comments on any distinctive odour of the breath and furring of the tongue.	0	1	2
8	Feels for lymphadenopathy in the neck and supraclavicular fossae.	0	1	2
9	Inspects the abdomen commenting on contour, asymmetry, distension, movement with breathing, scars, striae, spider naevi, visible veins and any visible masses, peristalsis or pulsations. Asks patient to lift their head looking for masses, hernias or sepration of muscles.	0	1	2
10	Asks if the patient has any pain in the abdomen and then gently palpates the abdomen superficially for masses, tenderness and muscular resistance (guarding) leaving the painful area until last. Follows an S-shaped pattern to ensure all quadrants are palpated.	0	1	2
11	Performs deep palpation following the same pattern.	0	1	2
12	Palpates for the liver with the radial edge of the index finger, asking the patient to take deep breaths. Percusses if an enlarged liver is felt.	0	1	2
13	Palpates for the spleen with the radial	0	1	2

	edge of the index finger, asking the patient to take deep breaths. Rolls patient towards their right side as the examining hand is gently worked up towards the left costal margin. Percusses if an enlarged spleen is felt and feels for the splenic notch.			
14	Palpates the right and the left kidney bimanually by placing one hand under the back and the other on the front of the loin. Asks patient to take a deep breath whilst balloting the kidney.	0	1	2
15	Palpates for the bladder in the hypogastric area and if a mass is palpable, percusses to confirm the presence of fluid.	0	1	2
16	Feel for the presence of an abdominal aortic aneurysm.	0	1	2
17	Checks for free fluid in the abdomen by performing shifting dullness and fluid thrill tests if the abdomen is distended.	0	1	2
18	Asks the patient to cough and inspects and feels for the presence of groin herniae.	0	1	2
19	Auscultates for bowel sounds.	0	1	2
20	States that they would complete the examination by carrying out a digital rectal examination.			
21	Thanks patient, asks them to dress and washes hands			

1. It is important to introduce yourself (give your name and what you do) and explain that you would like to examine their abdomen. Explain that you need to expose their abdomen fully in order to perform an adequate examination. Explain what you are going to do as you proceed with the examination, *before* you do it! A chaperone is essential for your own protection!
2. A general inspection provides an opportunity to assess whether the patient looks well or ill and to look around the bed for any clues to the diagnosis.
3. Tachycardia suggests that there may be infection or hypovolaemia (e.g. due to acute GI bleeding). Atrial fibrillation may throw off emboli into the mesenteric arteries, which can lead to bowel ischaemia with severe abdominal pain.
4. GI causes of clubbing include GI lymphoma, inflammatory bowel disease or coeliac disease.
   Koilonychia (spoon shaped nails) is indicative of anaemia.
   Leuconychia is opacification of the nail bed, which may be due to hypoalbuminaemia.
   Palmar erythema can be a sign of chronic liver disease (but can also be found in many other conditions or as a normal variant).
   Dupytren's contracture is a visible and palpable thickening and contraction of the palmar fascia causing permanent flexion, most often of the ring finger. It is associated with alcoholism but may also be found in manual workers or can be familial.

5. Liver flap is a coarse irregular tremor occurring when the arms are held outstretched with the wrists dorsiflexed (ask them to hold them there for 15 seconds). It occurs in liver failure.
   Excessive bruising may indicate that there is a clotting abnormality, which could be due to liver disease.
   Scratch marks suggest pruritis, which is a feature of cholestatic jaundice.
6. Pale conjunctivae are a sign of anaemia.
   Jaundice is best seen in the sclerae in natural light.
   Kayser-Fleischer rings are brownish green rings at the periphery of the cornea due to deposits of copper (as occurs in Wilson's disease, which causes cirrhosis).
7. Angular stomatitis refers to reddish brown cracks radiating from the corners of the mouth. Causes include vitamin B_6, B_{12}, folate and iron deficiency. It may be caused by infection in children.
   Circumoral pigmentation is one of the features of Peutz-Jeugers syndrome signifying underlying small bowel polyposis.
   Telangiectasiae may belie the existence of others elsewhere in the intestine (which can bleed).
   Glossitis refers to a smooth red appearance of the tongue. It is seen in B_{12} / folate deficiency (painful) and iron deficiency (painless).
   Aphthous ulcers may be due to inflammatory bowel disease, coeliac disease or can be idiopathic. Ulcers on the tongue may be malignant.
   Fetor hepaticus is a sweet-smelling odour on the breath, which occurs in severe hepatocellular disease. Alcohol and cigarette odours may also be detectable on the breath.
   Leukoplakia is white coloured thickening of the mucosa of the tongue and mouth, which may be premalignant. Candidiasis infection causes creamy white curd-like patches in the mouth and may spread to involve the oesophagus causing dysphagia.
8. It is particularly important to feel for lymph nodes in the left supraclavicular fossa (Virchow's nodes) in patients presenting with dysphagia as these drain lymph from the oesophagus. They may also become enlarged in advanced malignancy from anywhere in the upper GI tract. The presence of a large left supraclavicular node in association with carcinoma of the stomach is called Troisier's sign.
9. Contour is described as flat, rounded or scaphoid. Symmetry should be noted and any visible peristalsis observed. A distended abdomen may be due to fat, flatus, foetus, faeces or fluid. Local swellings may indicate enlargement of one of the abdominal or pelvic organs. It is important to note whether they move with, or independently of, respiration.
   The abdomen should move symmetrically with respiration and this is best assessed by squatting beside the bed so that the abdomen is at eye level. Asymmetrical movement indicates the presence of a mass. The abdomen will be still in peritonitis.
   Engorged veins may be visible. These are generally due to portal hypertension (where the characteristic caput medusae pattern occurs), or IVC obstruction (due to tumour, thrombosis or tense ascites).
   Scars are particularly important to note as they give information regarding previous surgery.
   Striae can be caused by ascites, pregnancy or recent loss of weight but also occur in Cushing's syndrome (here they are likely to be wider and purple-coloured).
   The presence of more than five spider naevi on the upper abdomen and chest is abnormal and may be related to cirrhosis.
   An expansile central pulsation in the epigastrum may be an abdominal aortic aneurysm. However, in very thin people, the abdominal aorta may be seen to pulsate normally.

Visible peristalsis may indicate pyloric obstruction (test for succussion splash) or obstruction of the distal small bowel (but may be a normal finding in very thin patients).

Lifting the head will tense the abdominal muscles and highlight any muscular weakness or defect and hernias. Masses within the abdominal wall should become more obvious.

10. Palpate each quadrant turn using the palmar surface of the fingers, moulding the hand to the shape of the abdominal wall. Watch the patient's face for any expression of pain or discomfort whilst palpating.

11. Deeper palpation allows detection of deeper masses and allows masses already discovered to be defined.

12. Palpation should begin in the right iliac fossa. A normal liver edge may be palpable just below the costal margin on deep inspiration in thin people. Causes of hepatomegaly include fatty infiltration, myeloproliferative disease, congestive cardiac failure, acute viral hepatitis, metastases or primary tumours.

    The liver span can be estimated by percussing down the right mid-clavicular line until liver dullness is encountered and measuring from there to the palpable liver edge.

    The gallbladder may be palpable, near the tip of the 9th costal cartilage, in carcinoma head of pancreas, mucocele of the gallbladder, carcinoma of the gallbladder or in acute cholecystitis. Courvoisier's law states that if the patient is jaundiced and the gallbladder is palpable, the cause is likely to be malignancy rather than gallstones.

13. Palpation for splenomegaly should also begin in the right iliac fossa. Place your left hand behind the left lower ribs and your right hand in the right iliac fossa and press the tips of your fingers asking the patient to take deep breaths. Work towards the left costal margin. Splenomegaly becomes detectable if the spleen is enlarged to twice or three times normal. Common causes include portal hypertension, leukaemia, lymphoma, haemolytic anaemia, some connective tissue disorders and infection e.g. malaria.

14. The lower pole of the right kidney may be palpable in thin normal persons. To distinguish a palpable kidney from the spleen, attempt to push your hand between it and the ribs (easy if the mass is renal), feel for the presence of a splenic notch, and try balloting the kidney bimanually.

    Causes of a unilateral palpable kidney include renal cell carcinoma, hydronephrosis, polycystic kidneys or renal abscesses. Bilateral palpable kidneys may be due to polycystic kidneys or bilateral hydronephrosis.

15. If there is urinary retention, a full bladder may be palpable above the pubic symphysis. It will be impossible to feel the lower border and the mass will be dull to percussion. Pressing on the area will make the patient uncomfortable and want to urinate.

16. The pulsation of an aortic aneurysm is expansile. If it is larger than 5 cm in diameter it warrants consideration for surgical repair.

17. When fluid accumulates in the abdomen, gravity causes it to collect in the flanks. If a dull percussion note suggesting fluid is detected in the flanks, the point where dullness is reached should be marked and the patient rolled onto their opposite side. If the area of dullness then becomes resonant it suggests that there is free fluid present.

    A fluid thrill is detected by asking the patient to place the edge of their palm firmly on the centre of the abdomen with the fingers pointing towards the groin. Flicking the side of the abdominal wall will cause a thrill to be felt by the examiner's hand placed on the other abdominal wall if there is massive ascites.

18. A hernia may be visible as an obvious swelling but may require the patient to bring it out by coughing. To fully examine a hernia, the patient must be standing.

19. Normal bowel sounds are heard intermittently all over the abdomen. Complete absence of bowel sounds over a 3 minute period suggests paralytic ileus. Bowel obstruction leads to louder, high pitch sounds with a tinkling quality.
20. A rectal examination is an important part of all GI examinations but will not be expected in an OSCE situation. If a mass is felt, it is important to assess whether it is arising from the rectal mucosa or is extrarectal. Causes of a palpable mass in the rectum include rectal carcinoma, rectal polyp, uterine or ovarian malignancy, prostatic or cervical malignancy, endometriosis and sigmoid colon carcinoma (prolapsing into the pouch of Douglas).
21. It is polite to thank the patient, inform them that the examination has concluded and that they may dress. Always wash your hands to reduce the risk of cross-infection.

Causes of Splenomegaly

CHICAGO:
Cancer
Haematological (PRV)
Infection
Congestion (portal hypertension)
Autoimmune (RA, SLE)
Glycogen storage disorders
Other (amyloidosis)

Causes of Ileus

MD SPUGERS:
Mesenteric ischemia
Drugs (see below)
Surgical (post-op)
Peritonitis/ Pancreatitis (sentinnel loop)
Unresolved mechanical obstruction (eg mass, intussusception, blockage)
Gram negative sepsis
Electrolyte imbalance (eg hypokalemia)
Retroperitoneal bleed or hematoma
Spinal or pelvic fracture
· Drugs are Aluminum hydroxide, Ba++, Ca carbonate, opiates, TCA, verapamil.

Digital Rectal Examination

		Not Attempted	Attempted inadequate	Attempted adequate
1.	Introduce self to patient and role	0	1	2
2.	Explain procedure and obtains verbal consent	0	1	2
3.	Washes hands and wear gloves	0	1	2
4.	Ensures examination area is private	0	1	2
5.	Asks for a chaperone	0	1	2
6.	Ensures bed height is appropriate	0	1	2
7.	Exposes patient appropriately	0	1	2
8.	Positions patient in left lateral position	0	1	2
9.	Parts buttocks and inspect (anal tags, candiasis, warts, fissures etc)	0	1	2
10.	Places gel on index finger and anus	0	1	2
11	Asks patient if there is any anal pain or if defecation is painful before inserting finger			
12	Warns patient and inserts finger, beginning using light pressure of the tip of the finger against the anus before advancing finger gently (consider the action of ringing a doorbell!)	0	1	2
13.	Examines anterior wall of rectum feeling for the prostate in men (size, shape, consistency – normally like a walnut!)	0	1	2
14.	Examine the rectum further for masses or faeces	0	1	2
15.	Ask patient to squeeze against finger to check anal tone	0	1	2
16.	On withdrawl check fingers for blood / pus / faeces	0	1	2
17	Proceeds to protoscopy or sigmoidoscope if necessary.			
18.	Wipes and cleans patient	0	1	2
19.	Disposes of gloves	0	1	2
19.	Allows them to dress	0	1	2
20.	Thanks patient	0	1	2
21.	Washes hands	0	1	2

1. It is polite to introduce yourself to the patient and what your role in their care is.
2. Rectal examination is an uncomfortable and embarrassing procedure for the patient. You should give a full explanation of the procedure and warn them that it can be uncomfortable.
3. Washing your hands and wearing well-fitting gloves is essential.
4. Ensuring privacy will calm and reassure the patient.
5. A chaperone is for your own protection!
6. This will save you having to bend down awkwardly.
7. Ideally, lower body garments should be removed.
8. This is for examination with the index finger of the right hand. Ask them to bend their knees upto their chest with their bottom facing you.
9. Inspection is essential. If a fissure is obviously visible, be very wary of hurting the patient.
10. Good lubrication is essential to a smooth examination.
11. Proceed with caution and gentleness if this is the case.
12. Warning the patient will stop them being startled and allow a smooth examination.
13-14. DRE can diagnose lower rectal cancers and prostate cancers.
15. This may be lax in the elderly or in women after a difficult vaginal delivery.
16. The presence of blood mandates a further examination of the recto-sigmoid colon with a sigmoidoscope. Pus may indicate an anal fistula or rectal crohn's disease.
17. This will depend on the DRE findings and is only necessary if a mucosal lesion is suspected.
18-21. It is polite to wipe the patient to allow them to dress without soiling their underclothes. Always wash and disinfect your hands after a rectal examination.

Examination of a Groin Hernia

		Not Attempted	Attempted inadequate	Attempted adequate
1.	Introduces self, explains role and gains consent	0	1	2
2.	Asks for chaperone and washes hands	0	1	2
3.	Ensures privacy	0	1	2
4	Exposes patient's groins adequately			
5	Asks patient where they feel the hernia is	0	1	2
6.	For groin hernias, examines patient standing up initially	0	1	2
7.	Inspects groins for scars and inspects for a lump asking patient to cough			
8	Assesses whether the scrotum and testes are normal and confirms that the bulge is coming from above the external ring	0	1	2
9.	Asks patient if it is tender, places hand on hernia and asks patient to cough. Attempts gently to push it back and asks patient to cough again	0	1	2
10.	Asks patient to lie down and reduces hernia gently. Checks if tender or irreducible. Notes whether hernia reduces with a gurgle	0	1	2
11.	Marks the pubic tubercle and the anterior superior iliac spine and calculates the approximate position of the internal inguinal ring	0	1	2
12.	Reduces hernia and presses on internal ring asking patient to cough again	0	1	2
13.	Differentiates between inguinal and femoral hernia by determining whether the lump is below and medial or above and lateral to the pubic tubercle	0	1	2
14	Thanks patient, asks them to dress and washes hands	0	1	2

1) It is important to introduce yourself (give your full name and role). Explain that you would like to examine their groins and gain verbal consent.

2) Asking for a chaperone protects you as a doctor from any possible accusations and is a must for both males and females. This can also reassure the patient.

3) Ensuring privacy is important to maintain patient dignity and helps the patient relax.

4) Appropriately expose the patient; it is best to remove trousers and pants and lift up shirt or top.

5) The patient will have presented with a lump, they may point to it which helps in the diagnosis.

6) This practice varies and it may be best to tell the examiner at this stage that you prefer to examine them standing up first and ask if that is OK. If the examiner says to start with patient lying down first, do this step at the end.

7) Inspection for scars will help determine whether the hernia is a recurrence of a previous repair. The appearance of a lump on coughing will help your diagnosis.

8) Examine the testes for any abnormal lumps and the upper part of the scrotum for an abnormal mass. Inguinoscrotal hernias descend through the inguinal canal into the scrotum.

9) Tenderness indicates obstruction or strangulation. If the hernia is tender and not easily reducible lie them down and attempt to reduce it again. If non-reducible, assess for small bowel obstruction.

10) Hernias which reduce with a gurgle contain bowel.

11) The internal inguinal ring lies 2/3^{rds} of the distance between the pubic tubercle and the anterior superior iliac spine

12) Pressure on the internal ring can usually block an indirect hernia from protruding

14) Conduct the examination in a fluent and professional manner. Always thanks the patient and wash your hands after each examination.

Differential diagnosis of inguinal lump
"**H**ernias **V**ery **M**uch **L**ike **T**o **S**well":   **H**ernias (inguinal, femoral)   **V**ascular (femoral aneurysm, sapheno varyx)   **M**uscle (psoas abscess)   **L**ymph nodes   **T**esticle (ectopic, undescended)   **S**permatic cord (lipoma, hydrocoele)

Examination Of A Patient With Acute Abdominal Pain

		Not attempted	Attempted inadequate	Attempted adequate
1	Approaches the patient politely and introduces him/herself. Exposes the patient from nipples to knees after obtaining their permission.	0	1	2
2	Feels the radial pulse, commenting on rate and regularity.	0	1	2
3	Looks at the eyes commenting on jaundice or pallor.	0	1	2
4	Looks with a torch around and inside the mouth. Comments on any distinctive odour of the breath and furring of the tongue.	0	1	2
5	Inspects the abdomen commenting on shape (especially distension), movement with breathing, scars, and any visible masses or pulsations.	0	1	2
6	Gently palpates the abdomen superficially for masses and tenderness, examining the sore area last. If the patient is 'sore all over', performs gentle superficial palpation to determine the presence of peritonitis.	0	1	2
7	If the soreness is localised to a part of the abdomen, gently determines whether there is guarding.	0	1	2
8	Examines for rebound tenderness.	0	1	2
9	Examines for percussion tenderness.	0	1	2
10	Asks the patient to cough or draw their abdomen in and blow it out. Enquires whether and where these movements cause pain.	0	1	2
11	If the pain is in the right upper quadrant, examines for 'Murphy's sign'.	0	1	2
12	Auscultates for bowel sounds.	0	1	2
13	Examines the hernial orifices.	0	1	2
14	Tells the examiner that a digital rectal examination and urinalysis are mandatory.	0	1	2
15	Thanks patient, asks them to dress and washes hands	0	1	2

1. It is important to introduce yourself (give your name and what you do) and explain that you would like to examine their abdomen. Explain that you need to expose their abdomen fully in order to perform an adequate examination. Explain what you are going to do as you proceed with the examination, *before* you do it! You must be very cautious when examining a patient with acute abdominal pain so as not to cause them further pain.

2. Tachycardia occurs with infection or hypovolaemia.

3. Jaundice with abdominal pain is usually due to gallstones.

4. Furring of the tongue and malodorous breath can occur with intra-abdominal sepsis (e.g. peritonitis or appendicitis).

5. Absence of abdominal wall movement with respiration suggests generalised peritonitis. A ruptured abdominal aortic aneurysm may form a visible expansile pulsation but often it will only be detected on palpation.

6. Localised abdominal pain is usually caused by inflammation of the underlying organ. Try to familiarise yourself with the surface anatomy of abdominal organs. Rigidity is constant involuntary contraction of the abdominal muscles resulting from peritoneal irritation.

7. Guarding refers to resistance to palpation caused by contraction of the abdominal muscles and may result from tenderness or anxiety.

8. Rebound tenderness is said to be present when there is a sudden pain when the abdomen is released rapidly after compression. This strongly suggests the presence of peritonitis. It can be uncomfortable for the patient so decide whether or not it is necessary before proceeding.

9. Tenderness to light percussion over the abdomen suggests peritonitis.

10. Coughing and movement worsen the pain of peritonitis.

11. Murphy's sign is positive if the patient catches his / her breath when taking a deep inspiration with the examiner's hand pressing just below the right costal margin. It is indicative of an inflamed gallbladder.

12. Bowel sounds will be 'tinkling' in intestinal obstruction and absent in peritonitis.

13. Small bowel can become strangulated in an inguinal hernia.

14. Note any tenderness or masses on rectal examination. The presence of blood may indicate acute colitis. Urinalysis may show haematuria in renal colic and glycosuria and ketonuria in diabetic ketoacidosis.

15. It is polite to thank the patient, inform them that the examination has concluded and that they may dress. Always wash your hands to reduce the risk of cross-infection.

Signs of Toxicity and Sepsis **6 T's:**
Tachycardia
Tachypnoea
Tremors
Toxic look
Tiredness
Temperature (fever)

Causes of acute pancreatitis

GET SMASH'D
- **G**allstones
- **E**thanol
- **T**rauma
- **S**teroids
- **M**umps,
- **A**utoimmune(PAN)
- **S**corpion bites
- **H**yperlipidemia,
- **D**rugs(azathioprine, diuretics)

Gastrointestinal Bleeding

		Not attempted	Attempted inadequate	Attempted adequate
1	Performs a preliminary assessment of airway, breathing and circulation. If profuse haemorrhage is occurring, asks for immediate help.	0	1	2
2	Washes hands and obtains intravenous access and sends bloods for FBC/U+E/LFTs/Clotting/Group and save or crossmatch.			
3	Asks the patient's name, DOB and occupation and introduces self and role	0	1	2
4	Asks whether the patient has vomited blood or passed it per rectum	0	1	2
5	Asks the amount and the colour of blood vomited (fresh red, clots or coffee ground). Distinguishes this from the coughing of blood (haemoptysis)	0	1	2
6	Asks the amount and colour of blood passed per rectum (fresh red and on toilet tissue or pan). Asks whether it was mixed with stool. Asks whether it was black and tarry. Asks if the patient is taking oral iron tablets. Distinguishes this from vaginal bleeding.			
7	Asks about history of dysphagia.	0	1	2
8	Asks about history of indigestion, heartburn or dyspepsia.	0	1	2
9	Takes a drug history and especially asks whether the patient is taking aspirin, non-steriodal analgesics, antiplatelet drugs or steroids.			
10	Asks about history of diarrhoea, constipation of a recent change in bowel habit.	0	1	2
11	Asks about history of passage of mucous and slime per rectum	0	1	2
12	Asks about weight loss and loss of appetite.	0	1	2
13	Asks about history of jaundice. Asks about previous history of liver disease and amount of alcohol intake.	0	1	2
14	Asks whether there is easy bruising and prolonged bleeding from minor cuts.			
15	Asks about past or current medical conditions, previous abdominal surgery and previous endoscopic examinations.	0	1	2
16	Asks about family history of bowel cancer or other bowel disorders.	0	1	2
17	Asks about home circumstances.	0	1	2
18	Asks about smoking.	0	1	2

1. For any patient with GI bleeding, it is important to initially assess whether immediate resuscitative measures are required. If the patient is haemodynamically unstable, hypotensive, tachycardic and hypoxic, immediate attention needs to be paid to that aspect of treatment first. If you are on your own, ask for help immediately.

2. Early intravenous access is important and more so if there is haemodynamic instability. At the same time, blood can be sent for tests and group and save (if no tachycardia or hypotension) and crossmatch 4 units (if patient is unstable)

3. Correctly identify the patient and it is polite to introduce yourself and your role in the management of the patient.

4. Vomiting of blood (haematemesis) usually originates in the oesophagus, stomach or duodenum. Passing altered blood per rectum (black and tarry) also originates in the upper digestive tract or right colon. Fresh red blood per rectum (haematochaezia) usually originates in the left colon, rectum and anus. Occasionally a profusely bleeding duodenal ulcer can cause fresh red rectal bleeding but this indicates exsanguinating blood loss.

5. This may give a clue to the cause and severity of the bleeding. Fresh blood with clots usually indicates a sizeable bleed which is continuing. 'Coffee ground' vomit is a slow bleed into the stomach and the appearance of the blood is altered by contact with gastric acid. It is important to ensure that the blood is not being coughed up as that has a completely different management pathway.

6. For rectal bleeding, blood mixed with stool usually originates in the rectum (usually cancer) and fresh red blood on the toilet tissue or pan usually indicates bleeding from piles. Black and tarry stools indicate bleeding higher up in the gastrointestinal tract (right colon, small bowel, duodenum, stomach or oesophagus). Oral iron tablets give the stool a silvery-back appearance. Elderly patients may sometimes not be able to distinguish between vaginal or rectal bleeding.

7. Oesophageal cancer and ulcers can cause dysphagia.

8. These are symptoms of oesophago-gastric and duodenal pathology.

9. Steroids and non-steroidal analgesics (NSAIDs) are a common cause of gastroduodenal ulceration. Antiplatelet drugs and aspirin can prevent the natural haemostatic mechanisms from working.

10,11. These are symptoms of colorectal pathology. Mucous and slime may indicate an inflammatory bowel disorder.

12. These are non-specific symptoms of malignant disease.

13. Liver cirrhosis can lead to oesophageal varices which can bleed.

14. These indicate a clotting disorder.
15. These may give clues to the site of the bleeding (e.g., diverticulitis).
16. Poor home circumstances can be associated with a higher risk of gastroduodenal ulceration and cancers.
17. Smoking increases the risk of ulcers and cancers of the gastrointestinal tract.

ALCOHOL HISTORY

		Not Attempted	Attempted inadequate	Attempted adequate
1.	Introduces him/herself to patient and obtains verbal consent	0	1	2
2.	Asks about presenting complaint and history of presenting complaint	0	1	2
3.	Asks patient whether they drink alcohol	0	1	2
4.	Assesses the pattern of drinking	0	1	2
5.	Establishes units per 24 hrs	0	1	2
6.	Establishes duration and trigger factors	0	1	2
7.	Establishes the effects of alcohol on his/her life	0	1	2
8.	Assesses dependency	0	1	2
9.	Assesses how the patient themselves views his/her alcohol intake	0	1	2
10.	Asks about other substance abuse	0	1	2
11.	Asks about family history of alcohol abuse	0	1	2
12.	Maintains good communication with the patient throughout without being judgemental	0	1	2

1) It is polite to introduce yourself, explain why you are there and get verbal consent from the patient.

2) Asking why the patient has come to hospital/clinic/ G.P. allows you to conduct a patient centered interview, addressing their problems before completing your questions.

3) Ask do you enjoy an alcoholic drink? This is a polite, non-judgemental way of opening the consultation.

4) Assess the patient's patterns of drinking. Do they drink every day? Do they binge drink? Do they drink at a particular time of day? Who do they drink with? Do they drink alone? Is there a particular reason why they drink e.g. to help with stress, boredom or to relax?

5) Ask about units per 24 hrs for an average day. At this stage you must clarify what they drink, ask specifically about beer/cider, wines and spirits, to ensure nothing is omitted from the history.

6) Assess how long they have been drinking to excess? Did anything cause an increase in their drinking? Does anything make them drink more? Ask about trigger factors, peer pressure, stress, and major life events.

7) Is alcohol affecting their life? **Social** - How do the patients family feel about his/her alcohol consumption. Has work been affected by this? Is their alcohol intake

affecting them financially? **Health** - Has the patient's health deteriorated since they've been drinking heavily? Have they been admitted to hospital due to alcohol? Things to think about with alcohol and the physical wellbeing of the patient; memory loss, pains, falls, headaches, vomiting, jaundice, pancreatitis, seizures, delirium tremens, Wernikoffs encephalopathy, G.I bleeding, ulcers and abnormal liver function tests.

Psychiatric wellbeing – Do they ever get low mood, depression, anxiety or see/hear things that other people don't see/hear (hallucinations)? Forensic History **– has alcohol ever got them into trouble with the law?**

8) There are various ways to assess dependency.

CAGE

Have you ever felt you should **C**UT down on your drinking?
Have people ever **A**NNOYED / ANGERED you by criticising your drinking?
Have you ever felt bad or **G**UILTY about your drinking?
Have you ever had a drink when you wake up in the morning to steady your nerves or get rid of a hangover? (**E**YE opener)

TWEAK

Do you have increased **T**olerance to alcohol?
Do you **W**orry about your alcohol consumption?
Do you ever have an **E**ye opener?
Have you ever had **A**mnesia after drinking?
Have you ever felt the need to **K**ut down on your drinking?
The TWEAK system uses a 7 points scoring, with 2 points for a positive score for **T** and **W** and 1 point for a positive score for **E**, **A** and **K**. More than or equal to 2 points suggests an alcohol problem.

9) Investigate the patient's view of their alcohol abuse. Do they see their drinking as a problem? Have they ever tried to stop drinking? (detoxing). Was this done with or without medical support? What was the end result? Do they want to cut down on their drinking and if so would they like medical help?
10) Ask about cigarettes and other illicit drugs.
11) Ask whether there is a family history of alcohol abuse or dependency. Alcoholism has a genetic predisposition.
12) Summarise back to patients appropriately.

The Cardiovascular System

General Cardiovascular History

		Not attempted	Attempted inadequate	Attempted adequate
1	Approaches the patient politely and introduces him/herself.	0	1	2
2	Asks the patient's name, DOB and occupation.	0	1	2
3	Asks about history of chest pain.	0	1	2
4	Asks about history of shortness of breath, orthopnoea and paroxysmal nocturnal dyspnoea.	0	1	2
5	Asks about history of palpitations.	0	1	2
6	Asks about history of ankle oedema.	0	1	2
7	Asks about history of syncope.	0	1	2
8	Asks about history of intermittent claudication.	0	1	2
9	Asks about history of fatigue.	0	1	2
10	Asks about relevant past or current conditions including hypertension, ischaemic heart disease, hypercholesterolaemia, rheumatic fever, diabetes, stroke and asthma.	0	1	2
11	Asks about family history of MI / stroke before the age of 65.	0	1	2
12	Asks about smoking and alcohol consumption.	0	1	2
13	Asks about home circumstances.	0	1	2
14	Asks about past and current medications, any allergies to medication and any previous surgery.	0	1	2

1. It is polite and professional to introduce yourself.

2. Name: to establish rapport and identify the patient.
   Age/DOB: certain diseases affect certain age groups, e.g. angina is rare in the under 40s. The DOB should be recorded to aid identifying the patient.
   Occupation: this can tell you a lot about the patient's background and can have significant effects on the management of their condition.

3. See specific history for chest pain.

4. Dyspnoea due to cardiac disease is typically chronic and insidious. The severity of dyspnoea can be gauged by asking about exercise tolerance. The presence of orthopnoea or PND implies that the underlying condition is probably cardiac rather than respiratory.

5. See specific history for palpitations.

6. Ankle oedema is a common symptom of right ventricular / congestive cardiac failure and is characteristically pitting, symmetrical and worse in the evenings.

In bed-bound patients, the oedema will be sacral rather than in the legs.

7. See specific history for syncope.

8. Patients with intermittent claudication complain of pain in their calves, thighs or buttocks which begins after walking a certain distance and is relieved by rest. It is a symptom of peripheral vascular disease.

9. Fatigue is a common symptom of cardiac failure but there are many other causes, which need to be excluded.
Drugs used for angina or hypertension, particularly β-blockers, can cause fatigue.

10. Patients with a history of previous angina or myocardial infarction are at risk of further cardiovascular and cerebrovascular events. Ask specifically what investigations have been carried out relating to these conditions in the past.
Hypertension, hypercholesterolaemia and diabetes are risk factors for ischaemic heart disease.
Rheumatic fever predisposes to valvular disease in later life.
Strokes can be due to ischaemic events in the cerebral circulation and are often associated with vascular disease elsewhere in the body.Asthma should be asked about because it contra-indicates the inclusion of β-blockers in the patient's management plan.

11. This is considered a positive family history and is an important risk factor for ischaemic heart disease.

12. Smoking is a risk factor for cardiovascular and peripheral vascular disease.
Heavy alcohol intake can lead to an alcoholic cardiomyopathy and is a risk factor for hypertension and cardiac arrhythmias.

13. Heart disease is a chronic condition, which severely reduces a patient's exercise tolerance and can be debilitating. Patients may be limited in their work and home environments and need to make adaptations.

14. It is necessary to establish which treatments, if any, have been tried previously and whether there were any adverse reactions.
Many drugs are capable of inducing arrhythmias.
Anti-hypertensive medications can cause postural hypotension which may lead to syncope. In the case of a patient presenting with an MI, specifically ask about any recent surgery as it may be a contra-indication to thrombolysis.

Presenting Complaint - Chest Pain

		Not attempted	Attempted inadequate	Attempted adequate
1	Asks the patient to point to the site where the pain is worst.	0	1	2
2	Asks whether the pain radiates anywhere else.	0	1	2
3	Asks the patient to describe the character of the pain.	0	1	2
4	Asks about the onset and duration of the pain.	0	1	2
5	Asks whether the pain is constant or intermittent.	0	1	2
6	Asks whether anything makes the pain better or worse.	0	1	2
7	Asks the patient to rate the severity of the pain.	0	1	2
8	Asks whether the patient has ever had anything like this before.	0	1	2
9	Asks whether the patient has noticed any ankle or leg swelling.	0	1	2
10	Asks whether the patient has any associated symptoms, specifically nausea, sweating, anxiety, cough or dyspnoea.	0	1	2
11	Asks specifically about risk factors for an MI (family history, hypertension, diabetes mellitus, smoking and hypercholesterolaemia).	0	1	2
12	Asks about previous history of DVT / PE and about any history of recent surgery, immobility, malignancy or pregnancy.	0	1	2
13	Asks about past and current medications.	0	1	2

1. Cardiac pain is usually central and crushing.
   Pain due to GOR, aortic dissection or pericarditis can all also be central but are distinguished from cardiac pain by their other features.
   Chest wall pain (e.g. due to muscle strain, rib fractures, thoracic nerve compression or thoracic herpes zoster) is typically well localised.
   The pain of a pneumothorax is also usually localised.

2. Cardiac pain typically radiates to the left arm, neck and / or jaw and occasionally into the teeth, back or abdomen.
   A dissecting aortic aneurysm causes pain that radiates to the back.
   Diseases of the cervical or upper thoracic spine cause pain that radiates from the back to the front of the chest.

3. A patient with angina may well feel 'discomfort' rather than pain, describing it as crushing, dull or aching in character. They may experience heaviness or paraesthesiae in one or both arms.

A myocardial infarction produces similar pain but it is usually more severe. Pleuritic pain, chest wall pain and the pain of a pneumothorax are characteristically sharp and severe.
A dissecting aortic aneurysm produces pain often described as 'tearing'.
A massive PE can cause either an angina type pain or a pleuritic pain and needs to be considered in context of the other features.
Oesophageal spasm and GOR are associated with heartburn and dysphagia.

4. Ischaemic pain that persists for more than 30 minutes is likely to be associated with damage to the heart muscle.
    Pain due to a massive PE, pneumothorax or dissecting aortic aneurysm is usually of sudden onset.

5. Pain that is associated with exertion, respiration or specific movements may be described by the patient as intermittent. Ask about the specific situations in which it occurs.

6. Angina is normally brought on by exertion and relieved by rest (angina occurring at rest is known as unstable angina). Nitrates tend to relieve the pain but this is not specific since nitrates will also relieve the pain of oesophageal spasm. Pleuritic pain is made worse by inspiration and is usually relieved by sitting up and leaning forwards.
    Chest wall pain is made worse by respiration or movement of the shoulders.
    Oesophageal spasm may be precipitated by drinking hot or cold fluids and is relieved by nitrates.

7. Severity is obviously subjective but someone who is used to angina pain will often report the pain of an MI to be more severe (beware diabetics and the elderly who may have 'silent' MIs).

8. If the patient is known to have angina, find out how it is managed, what investigations have been done previously and whether this episode is different in any way.

9. Unilateral leg swelling suggests that there may be a DVT and PE should therefore be one of the top differential causes for the chest pain.
    Many patients with mild degrees of heart failure will report ankle swelling but this will usually be bilateral and worse in the evenings.

10. MI often produces dyspnoea, sweating, anxiety, nausea and faintness in association with the chest pain. Pleuritic pain may be associated with symptoms of chest infection such as a productive cough and pyrexia. PEs can cause pain associated with dyspnoea and cough / haemoptysis. A pneumothorax produces dyspnoea as well as chest pain. Oesophageal spasm is associated with dysphagia.

11. It is essential to ask about these risk factors and to document the responses clearly in the notes.

12. Surgery, immobility, malignancy and pregnancy are all risk factors for DVTs.

13. The combined oral contraceptive pill increases the chances of a DVT / PE developing. If a patient had had a previous MI, ask if they were given thrombolysis as streptokinase should not be used twice.

Basic Management of MI
BOOMAR: **B**ed rest   **O**xygen   **O**piate   **M**onitor   **A**nticoagulate   **R**educe clot size

Presenting Complaint – Palpitations

		Not attempted	Attempted inadequate	Attempted adequate
1	Asks the patient to describe what they mean by palpitations.	0	1	2
2	Asks them to tap out the rate and rhythm of the palpitations.	0	1	2
3	Asks whether the palpitations are sudden in onset and how long they last.	0	1	2
4	Asks whether there is anything in particular that sets the palpitations off.	0	1	2
5	Asks whether there is anything that the patient can do to stop the palpitations e.g. holding their breath or coughing.	0	1	2
6	Asks whether there are any associated features, such as chest pain, fainting or breathlessness.	0	1	2
7	Asks whether the patient has any history of cardiac problems or hypertension.	0	1	2
8	Asks whether the patient has noticed any weight loss, heat intolerance, increased stool frequency or irritability recently.	0	1	2
9	Asks whether the patient has been feeling anxious recently or if they are under any unusual stress.	0	1	2
10	Asks about smoking and alcohol use.	0	1	2
11	Asks if the patient is on any medications.	0	1	2

1. Palpitations are defined as unexpected awareness of the heartbeat.

2. Note the rate and rhythm.
   An irregularly irregular heartbeat suggests atrial fibrillation.

3. Cardiac arrhythmias are sudden in onset whereas sinus tachycardia is usually insidious.

4. Patients may notice that they get palpitations when they are in anxiety provoking situations.
   Ectopic beats are more noticeable when the background rate is slow such as when the person is resting.
   Paroxysmal tachycardias are often precipitated by exercise or specific movements.
   Coffee, tea and alcohol are known to act as triggers in certain people.

5. Many patients may have found that coughing or swallowing terminates the palpitation (the Valsalva manoeuvre may terminate supraventricular tachycardia).

6. Sudden onset, rapid palpitations followed by syncope suggest ventricular tachycardia.
   Any rapid rhythm may precipitate angina in a patient with ischaemic heart disease.

7. MI, valvular disease cardiomyopathy, myocarditis and aberrant conduction pathways can cause arrhythmias, which may present as palpitations. Hypertensive patients are at increased risk of developing atrial fibrillation.

8. These are symptoms of thyrotoxicosis, which can cause palpitations.

9. Palpitations are one of the physical manifestations of anxiety.

10. Smoking is a risk factor for ischaemic heart disease and hypertension. Chronic alcohol excess can cause cardiomyopathy, which is associated with arrhythmias.

11. Find out if the patient is on any antiarrhythmic agents already and if so, whether they have been compliant.
    Many drugs are capable of causing arrhythmias, particularly in overdose.

Presenting Complaint – Intermittent Claudication

		Not attempted	Attempted inadequate	Attempted adequate
1	Asks the patient to describe the problem.	0	1	2
2	Asks where in the legs the pain is.	0	1	2
3	Asks them how far they have to walk before they get the pain.	0	1	2
4	Asks whether this distance is staying the same or decreasing.	0	1	2
5	Asks how long they have to rest for before the pain eases.	0	1	2
6	Asks whether they ever get pain at rest, particularly at night.	0	1	2
7	Asks whether bending forwards relieves the pain.	0	1	2
8	Asks whether the patient ever gets back pain or weakness, tingling or numbness in their legs.	0	1	2
9	Asks whether the patient suffers from impotence.	0	1	2
10	Asks whether they have noticed any skin changes in their legs.	0	1	2
11	Asks about risk factors for vascular disease including hypertension, high cholesterol, diabetes, smoking and family history.	0	1	2
12	Asks about any history of angina, MI or strokes.	0	1	2

1. Intermittent claudication is characterised by cramp-like pain in the legs on exercise, occurring after a certain distance and settling on rest after a certain time.

2. Calf pain signifies disease in the superficial femoral artery.
   Thigh pain signifies disease in the external iliac artery.
   Buttock pain signifies disease in the lower aorta or common and internal iliac arteries.

3. Claudication distance is an important indicator of the severity of the arterial disease.

4. The rate of progression of the condition is one of the factors determining the necessity for intervention.

5. As the arterial disease worsens, the pain will take longer to ease off.

6. Rest pain is a bad prognostic sign denoting chronic critical ischaemia which needs attention.
   Rest pain typically occurs at night and is relieved by hanging the foot over the side of the bed.

7. Spinal canal stenosis in the lumbar region causes pain in a root distribution brought on by walking and relieved by rest. It is important therefore to distinguish this from intermittent claudication. The pain of spinal canal stenosis is associated with neurological symptoms and is relieved by bending forwards as this opens up the spinal canal.

8. If the patient has back pain or neurological symptoms in the legs, it is likely that the leg pain is due to nerve root compression rather than to arterial disease.

9. Severe disease in the distal aorta can cause impotence in association with thigh claudication (the Leriche syndrome).

10. Chronically ischaemic legs are typically hairless with dry skin and, in severe cases, ulcers may develop.

11. The risk factors for peripheral vascular disease are the same as those for cardiovascular disease.

12. A history of ischaemic heart disease or strokes in a patient presenting with intermittent claudication suggest widespread arterial disease is present.

Causes of Raynaud's Disease

BAD CT:
Blood disorders (eg polycythaemia)
Arterial (eg atherosclerosis, Buerger's)
Drugs (eg beta-blockers)
Connective tissue disorders (rheumatoid arthritis, SLE, CREST)
Traumatic (eg vibration injury)

General Cardiovascular Examination

		Not attempted	Attempted inadequate	Attempted adequate
1	Approaches the patient politely and introduces him/herself. Positions the patient at 45°. Exposes the patient adequately after obtaining their permission.	0	1	2
2	Inspects the patient and their surrounds commenting on general appearance.	0	1	2
3	Examines the hands and nails, commenting on colour, clubbing, koilonychia, splinter haemorrhages, Osler's nodes, Janeway lesions and tendon xanthomas.	0	1	2
4	Feels for radial pulse. Comments on rate and rhythm.	0	1	2
5	Feels for a collapsing pulse by elevating the arm after first confirming that the patient has no pain in their shoulder.	0	1	2
6	Feels for radial-radial and radial-femoral delay.	0	1	2
7	Measures the blood pressure.	0	1	2
8	Examines the sclerae, conjunctivae and around the eyes, commenting on jaundice, pallor, xanthelasma and malar flush.	0	1	2
9	Looks inside the mouth, commenting on cyanosis, petechiae and tooth decay.	0	1	2
10	Assesses the JVP.	0	1	2
11	Feels the carotid pulse, commenting on its character.	0	1	2
12	Inspects the precordium commenting on scars or deformity and palpates the apex beat, commenting on any displacement.	0	1	2
13	Feels for parasternal impulses or thrills.	0	1	2
14	Auscultates over mitral, aortic, pulmonary and tricuspid areas. Comments on intensity, splitting, any added heart sounds or murmurs.	0	1	2
15	Sits the patient forward and inspects the back, commenting on scars or deformity.	0	1	2
16	Percusses and auscultates the lung bases.	0	1	2
17	Feels for sacral oedema.	0	1	2
18	Feels for ankle oedema and calf tenderness as well as commenting on signs of peripheral vascular disease.	0	1	2
19	Feels dorsalis pedis, posterior tibial, popliteal and femoral pulses on both sides.	0	1	2
20	Thanks patient, asks them to dress and washes hands	0	1	2

1. It is important to introduce yourself (give your name and what you do) and explain that you would like to examine their chest. Explain that you need to expose their chest and neck fully in order to perform an adequate examination. Respect the modesty of patients. Explain what you are going to do as you proceed with the examination, *before* you do it!

2. Decide whether the patient looks distressed or ill by considering their colour and respiratory pattern. There may be clues around the bedside such as oxygen or GTN spray.
   Cachexia (severe loss of weight and muscle wasting) often signifies malignancy but may occur in severe cardiac failure.
   Marfan's syndrome is associated with aortic regurgitation.
   Down's syndrome is associated with congenital heart disease.
   Turner's syndrome is associated with coarctation of the aorta.

3. Cardiovascular causes of clubbing include cyanotic congenital heart disease and subacute infective endocarditis.
   Splinter haemorrhages may be caused by infective endocarditis or profound anaemia.
   Koilonychia is a sign of iron deficiency anaemia, which may exacerbate angina.
   Osler's nodes are painful erythematous lumps in pulps of fingers and toes or the palms or soles. They are thought to be fragments of vegetation from an infected valve.
   Janeway lesions are non-tender erythematous maculopapular lesions containing bacteria in the palms or pulps of fingers of patients with infective endocarditis.
   Tendon xanthomata are yellow deposits of lipid in tendons, which occur in type II hyperlipidaemia.

4. If the pulse is irregular, decide whether it is regularly or irregularly irregular. The most common cause of an irregularly irregular pulse is atrial fibrillation.

5. A collapsing pulse (rapid upstroke and descent) occurs in aortic regurgitation, patent ductus arteriosus, or in a hyperdynamic circulation.

6. Radial - radial inequality in timing or volume suggests large arterial occlusion (atherosclerotic plaque or aneurysm).
   Radial-femoral delay suggests coarctation of the aorta.

7. The blood pressure should be checked both lying and standing to test for postural hypotension.

8. Jaundice may be caused by prosthetic heart valve induced haemolysis.
   Pallor is a sign of anaemia.
   Petechial haemorrhages in the conjunctivae may be due to embolic phenomena.
   Xanthelasma (yellow cholesterol deposits around eyes) may be a normal variant or may indicate hyperlipidaemia.
   A malar flush (rosy cheeks with a bluish tinge) may be due to dilatation of the malar capillaries associated with pulmonary hypertension and a low cardiac output (as occurs in severe mitral stenosis).

9. The tongue and lips are the best places to see central cyanosis.
Mucosal petechiae are a sign of infective endocarditis and dental caries may be the source of the responsible organisms.
A high arched palate occurs in Marfan's syndrome (see point 2).

10. The JVP is best assessed from the internal jugular vein, medial to sternomastoid.

To distinguish the JVP from the arterial pulse, the JVP:
- is a double impulse (a and v waves).
- varies with position and inspiration.
- cannot be palpated.
- rises transiently if pressure is applied over the liver.

The sternal angle is taken as the zero point and the maximum height of pulsation is given in cm above this. It should be <3cm (i.e. not above clavicle) when the patient is positioned at 45°.
An increased JVP can be caused by right ventricular failure, tricuspid stenosis or regurgitation, pericardial effusion, constrictive pericarditis, SVC obstruction or fluid overload.

11. The carotid pulse is palpable medial to sternomastoid at the level of the thyroid cartilage. Never palpate both carotid pulses together.

The pulse character is best assessed here:
- Slow rising in aortic stenosis.
- Collapsing in aortic regurgitation, a hyperdynamic circulation and patent ductus arteriosus.
- Bisferiens pulse is a combination of the slow rising and collapsing pulses occurring when aortic stenosis and incompetence are present together.
- A small volume pulse is a sign of aortic stenosis or pericardial effusion.
- Pulsus alternans refers to alternating weak and strong beats as occurs when the LV is severely diseased.

12. -14. See section on examination of the precordium.

15. Scars on the back are most likely due to trauma or operations on the lungs but they may provide important information regarding the patient's past medical history.

16. In cardiac failure late or pan-inspiratory crackles or a pleural effusion may be present.

17. Pitting oedema of the sacrum occurs in severe right heart failure, especially in patients who have been lying in bed.

18. Cardiac causes of bilateral lower limb oedema include congestive cardiac failure and constrictive pericarditis.
Unilateral lower limb oedema can be due to DVT or compression of large veins by tumour or lymph nodes. Note the upper level of the oedema.
Ischaemic legs are generally pulseless, pale, painful, paralysed and perishingly cold. They may also be ulcerated or gangrenous.

19. Dorsalis pedis - lateral to extensor hallucis longus tendon, proximal to 1st metatarsal space.

Posterior tibial - behind the medial malleolus.
Popliteal - the knee joint must be flexed and relaxed. Place both hands over the knee so your fingers are in the popliteal fossa on each side. Lift up quite firmly and feel for the pulse against the tibia.
Femoral - in the groin crease directly below the mid-inguinal point (midway between anterior superior iliac spine and the pubic symphysis).

20. It is polite to thank the patient, inform them that the examination has concluded and that they may dress. Always wash your hands to reduce the risk of cross-infection.

Causes of raised JVP

HOLT:
Heart failure
Obstruction of vena cava
Lymph node enlargement - supraclavicular
Thoracic pressure increase

Beck's Triad (Cardiac Tamponade)

3 D's
Distant heart sounds
Distended jugular veins
Decreased arterial pressure

Examination Of The Precordium

		Not attempted	Attempted inadequate	Attempted adequate
1	Inspects the precordium commenting on scars, any pacemaker box, skeletal deformity or visible pulsations.	0	1	2
2	Palpates for the apex beat (placing them in the left lateral position if necessary), a parasternal heave and thrills.	0	1	2
3	Auscultates over the mitral area (corresponds to the apex beat), thumb on neck in order to time the cycle with the carotid pulse.	0	1	2
4	Auscultates over the tricuspid area (just to the left of the lower sternum), thumb on neck.	0	1	2
5	Auscultates over the pulmonary area (2nd left intercostal space), thumb on neck.	0	1	2
6	Auscultates over the aortic area (2nd right intercostal space), thumb on neck.	0	1	2
7	Asks the patient to lie on their left side and auscultates over the mitral area and into the axilla.	0	1	2
8	Asks the patient to sit forward and hold their breath in full expiration whilst the examiner auscultates over the aortic area.	0	1	2
9	Comments on intensity and any splitting of the heart sounds at each position and any added sounds heard.	0	1	2
10	Describes any murmurs by their site, timing and radiation.	0	1	2
11	Listens for carotid bruits.	0	1	2
12	Thanks patient and washes hands			

1. The position of a scar can suggest whether the patient has had a CABG or a valve replacement.
Skeletal abnormalities may be part of Marfan's syndrome or may just be the normal anatomy for that person. They can distort the position of the heart and vessels in the chest causing displacement of the apex beat. If there is severe deformity, pulmonary function may be affected and pulmonary hypertension may result.
Pacemaker boxes are usually under the left pectoral muscle and easily palpable. The apex beat is sometimes visible as a pulsation. If there is severe pulmonary hypertension, there may be a visible pulsation over the pulmonary artery.

2. The apex beat normally lies in the 5th left intercostal space, 1cm medial to midclavicular line. It is displaced laterally and has a thrusting quality when there is volume overload, as in mitral or aortic regurgitation. It has a heaving quality but is not displaced in a pressure overloaded system (aortic stenosis).

When the patient is in the left lateral position, the apex of the heart is brought closer to the chest wall and the apex beat can be felt more easily.

Causes of an impalpable apex beat are DOPEE (dextrocardia, obesity, pneumothorax, emphysema and effusion).

Parasternal heaves are felt with the heel of the hand resting to the left of the sternum with the fingers lifted slightly off the chest. They occur when there is RV enlargement or severe LA enlargement.

Thrills are palpable murmurs felt with the flat of the hand. They should be felt for systematically over the apex, left sternal edge and then the base of the heart.

3-6. Palpation of the carotid pulse simultaneously with auscultation allows determination of which heart sound is which and allows any murmurs and added sounds to be timed.

Right sided heart murmurs are loudest in inspiration, when venous return is increased. Murmurs arising from the left side of the heart are loudest in expiration.

7. If the patient is turned towards their left side, sounds from the mitral valve are heard more clearly. Listen round into the axilla for the radiation of a mitral regurgitation murmur.

8. Leaning the patient forwards and listening whilst they are in full expiration allows better detection of aortic regurgitation.

9. The intensity of heart sounds is significant only when considered in relation to all other features of the case:
   - M_1 - loud in mitral stenosis.
   - A_2 / P_2 - loud in systemic / pulmonary hypertension and soft in aortic / pulmonary stenosis.

   Splitting of heart sounds:
   - Splitting of S_1 is difficult to hear. If it does occur, it is most commonly due to RBBB.
   - A_2 and P_2 are more widely separated. A_2 is heard in all areas whereas P_2 is normally only heard in the pulmonary area.
   - Normally P_2 follows A_2 and the splitting is widest in inspiration (RV stroke volume increases whereas LV stroke volume falls). Increased splitting occurs in RBBB, pulmonary stenosis and if there is a VSD.
   - Reverse splitting (P_2 heard first in expiration) occurs when LV emptying is delayed eg. in LBBB, aortic stenosis or coarctation of the aorta.

   3rd and 4th sounds:
   - Are lower frequency sounds heard in diastole.
   - A 3rd sound occurs in early diastole at the time of most rapid filling. It may occur in healthy young adults and in pregnancy but other than this is indicates abnormal LV filling (mitral regurgitation or LV failure).
   - A 4th sound occurs as the atria contract (only occurs in sinus rhythm). It is due to non-compliant ventricles or atrial hypertrophy (systemic hypertension) and is never physiological.
   - If the heart rate is rapid, diastole is shortened and the 3rd and 4th sounds coincide producing a gallop rhythm.

Additional sounds:
- Ejection systolic clicks are due to opening of semi-lunar valves and occur in early systole.
- Opening snaps of the mitral and tricuspid valves may be heard in mitral or tricuspid stenosis (usually followed by diastolic murmur).
- Mid-systolic clicks are associated with prolapse of the mitral valve.

10. Timing:
- Pansystolic - between the 1st and 2nd heart sounds. It occurs in mitral or tricuspid regurgitation and VSD.
- Ejection systolic - a crescendo - decrescendo murmur, peaking in mid-systole. It arises from the pulmonary or aortic outflow tracts.
- Late systolic - clear gap between 1st sound and the murmur. It occurs in mitral valve prolapse or mild mitral regurgitation.
- Early diastolic - short gap between S_2 and the beginning of the murmur. It occurs in aortic / pulmonary regurgitation.

Radiation:
- Aortic ejection murmurs radiate to the carotids.
- Aortic incompetence murmurs radiate to the left sternal edge.
- Mitral incompetence murmurs radiate to the mid-axillary line.

Mitral stenosis → opening snap (following S2) and then a low pitched rumbling mid-diastolic murmur, best heard at the apex. Providing the patient is not in atrial fibrillation, there will be a pre-systolic accentuation of the murmur.

Mitral regurgitation → soft S1 and then a pan-systolic murmur, loudest at the apex and radiating to the axilla. S3 may be audible.

Aortic stenosis → ejection click followed by an ejection systolic murmur, loudest in the aortic area and radiating to the carotids.

Aortic regurgitation → high pitched early diastolic murmur best heard at the left sternal edge. There is often also an ejection systolic murmur due to volume overload.

11. A carotid bruit indicates a narrowing of the carotid artery. They are easiest to hear if the patient holds their breath in inspiration. If a bilateral bruit is heard, be aware that it may be the radiation of the murmur of aortic stenosis.
12. It is good practice to wash and disinfect your hands after each examination to reduce the risk of cross-infection.

Description of a murmur

"IL PQRST" (person has ill PQRST heart waves):
Intensity
Location
Pitch
Quality
Radiation
Shape
Timing

Causes of Pericarditis

CARDIAC RIND:
Collagen vascular disease
Aortic aneurysm
Radiation
Drugs (such as hydralazine)
Infections
Acute renal failure
Cardiac infarction
Rheumatic fever
Injury
Neoplasms
Dressler's syndrome

Causes of impalpable apex beat
COPD
COPD
Obesity
Pleural, Pericardial effusion
Dextrocardia

Peripheral Vascular Examination

		Not Attempted	Attempted inadequate	Attempted adequate
1.	Introduces self to patient	0	1	2
2.	Explains examination and obtains consent	0	1	2
3.	Washes hands	0	1	2
4.	Correctly positions patient	0	1	2
5.	Adequately exposes patient	0	1	2
6.	Inspects lower limbs	0	1	2
7.	Feels temperature of the limbs	0	1	2
8.	Checks capillary refill	0	1	2
9.	Checks for pitting oedema	0	1	2
10.	Palpates lower limb pulses	0	1	2
11.	Auscultates for femoral bruits	0	1	2
12.	Checks for presence of AAA (abdominal aortic aneurysm)	0	1	2
13.	Mentions/performs: Buerger's test Trendelenburg test Ankle/Brachial Pressure Index (ABPI)	0	1	2
14.	Inspects upper limbs	0	1	2
15.	Takes the radial pulse, check for radial-radial delay and radial femoral delay	0	1	2
16.	Feels for the ulnar, bracial and carotid pulses.			
17.	Mentions Blood pressure	0	1	2
18.	Listens for carotid bruits	0	1	2
19.	Mentions / performs Allen's test	0	1	2
20.	Thank the patient and allows them to get dressed	0	1	2
21.	Washes hands and documents the findings	0	1	2

1) It is both polite, rapport building and necessary to greet a patient and confirm their identity. It is important the patient knows both who you are and what your role is.
2) Explain the procedure so the patient knows what to expect and what is required of them. This may help put them at ease and make your job easier. Obtain verbal consent.
3) Hand washing is vital to prevent the spread of infections.
4) Position - patient should be lying in the supine position. The patient's hands should remain at their sides with their head resting on a pillow.
5) Ensure patient's legs and arms are exposed. Cover the patient with a blanket to maintain their modesty when you are not examining them.

6) Inspect for:-
- Signs of trauma / scarring (previous surgery - especially graft sites).
- Erythema (redness).
- Look for symmetry between limbs.
- Skin changes - hair loss or shiny this skin indicates PVD
- Look at colour of the limb – well perfused / cyanosed?
- Pigmentation
- Oedema
- Varicose veins
- Muscle wasting
- Ulcers – arterial / neuropathic / venous.

Palpation
7) Feel the temperature of limbs - cool suggests poor circulation. Compare like with like. (A unilateral red hot swollen limb may be due to a DVT (deep venous thrombosis)
8) Capillary refill is the rate at which blood refills empty capillaries. It can be measured by pressing a fingernail for 4-5 seconds until it turns white, and taking note of the time needed for color to return once the nail is released. Normal refill time is less than 2 seconds. This is a measures of perfusion.
9) Check for pitting oedema – press down over bony area of the shins.
10) Palpate arterial Pulses – are they present?

Dorsalis pedis – dorsal surface of the foot – between the 1st and 2nd metatarsals running laterally to the tendon.
Posterior tibial – posterior to the medial malleolus
Popliteal – behind the knee, between the heads of the gastronaemus muscles. Palpate with BOTH hands.
Femoral – halfway between the pubic symphisis and anterior superior iliac spine.

Auscultate
11) Femoral bruits – caused by turbulent flow due to a blockage/narrowing. They sound like a rushing noise (like listening to the sea!)

12) Feel for the presence of abdominal aortic aneurysm. They are most common in men who smoke and are over 60. The aorta lies at the midline of the abdomen. Place both hands flat on the patient's abdomen, thumbs touching with one hand either side on the midline. Carefully feel for an abnormally wide pulsation. Note that even large aneurysms can be very difficult to detect on physical examination

13) Specific Tests
- Burgers sign – raise legs 45 degrees for 2mins – then ask patient to swing legs over the edge of the bed – white soles on raising the legs indicates ischaemia the arterial supply is not greater than gravity. Most patients will quickly turn pink, but a red colour upon reperfusion indicated ischaemia. (i.e., blue then red is a positive test)
- Trendelenburg test - Used to assess varicose veins if present. Take one leg at a time. With the patient supine, empty the superficial veins by milking the leg distally to proximally. Press down using thumb over the saphenofemoral junction (2cm below and 2cm lateral to pubic tubercle), maintain pressure while the patient stands. If the leg refills, the incompetence is below the junction.

- Mention Ankle Brachial Pressure Index (ABPI). The test assesses PVD (peripheral vascular disease) and is a measure of the fall in blood pressure in the arteries supplying the legs. A reduced ABPI (less than 0.8) is consistent with PVD.

<u>Upper Body</u>
14) Inspect – same as with the lower limb.
15) Take the radial pulse. Comment on rate (beats per minute), whether it is regular or irregular and the character (normal, bounding, weak, slow rising etc). Compare pulses for radial – radial delay (occlusion or aortic stenosis) and radial - femoral delay (coactation of the aorta or occlusion).
16) Check the other peripheral pulses, the ulnar, brachial and carotid.
17) Mention blood pressure.
18) Listen for carotid bruits
19) ALLEN's Test:- Elevate the patient's hand and ask them to make a fist for 30 seconds. Put pressure over both the radial and ulnar arteries, occluding them. With the hand still elevated, ask the patient to open their hand (it should appear blanched). Release the ulnar artery and look for the colour returning (within 7 seconds). If the colour does not return in 7 second then the ulnar circulation is insufficient. Repeat test with the radial artery.
20) This is polite
21) Always wash your hands and document the findings while they are fresh in your memory.

Top Tips

Electrocardiography (ECG)

ECG Lead Placement

ECG electrodes comprise of 12 leads which are placed on the limbs and precordium in the following manner:

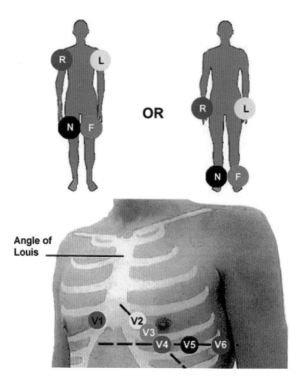

Angle of Louis

V1: Fourth intercostal space to the right of the sternum.
V2: Fourth intercostal space to the Left of the sternum.
V3: Directly between leads V2 and V4.
V4: Fifth intercostal space at midclavicular line.
V5: Level with V4 at left anterior axillary line.
V6: Level with V5 at left midaxillary line.
(Directly under the midpoint of the armpit)

Understanding ECGs

An ECG is a two dimensional recording of a three dimensional process. A cardiac electrical impulse does not travel in a single direction down a straight line with an arrow on the end. It in fact spreads out in all directions across the heart. The ECG leads allow us to look at this depolarisation wave from different views--that is, in the vertical and horizontal planes. When the wave is heading towards a specific lead we will get the largest positive deflection in that lead. When it is heading directly away from it we will get the opposite: the largest negative response. Leads looking at right angles to the wave front will see smaller biphasic responses as the wave passes them. We will go through the different parts that make up the ECG recording (see figure 1) in turn.

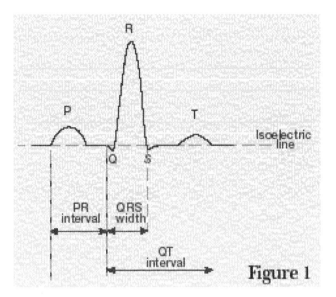

Figure 1

The P-wave

This is a recording of atrial depolarisation. Most of the time this starts in the sinoatrial (SA) node and the predominant direction of the impulse across the atria is inferiorly and from right to left. This generates a positive deflection in the leads that look at the heart from below. (See figure 2.) As five of the six chest leads are mostly on the left side of the body and in approximately the same vertical plane there will generally not be much difference in the P-wave in these leads with small positive deflections seen in each. Lead V1 looks across the atria and sees the atrial depolarisation pass across its view. Thus the P-wave typically has a biphasic waveform in this particular lead. As we have said before, the chest leads are not good at looking at vertical movement. As one of the predominant movements of this depolarisation is downwards (inferiorly), then the chest leads do not detect this well, apart from lead V1 with its different view on the heart.

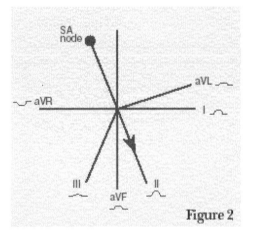

Figure 2

Occasionally, if there is damage to the SA node, the initiation of the electrical activity can arise from other parts of the atria. If this is lower down in the atria the impulse has to move in the opposite direction to normal. In these circumstances P-wave deflections are in the opposite direction. (See figure 3.) We point this out, not because it is common or particularly important, but because it is a simple example of seeing what the different leads record in changing circumstances.

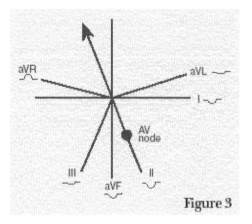

Figure 3

Key facts about P-wave

- Initiated at SA node

- Predominantly travels inferiorly and from right to left in the normal individual

- The rate of firing of the SA node normally determines the heart rate

- Limb lead II is the lead that normally best shows the P-wave, and lead V1 provides an alternative view

- The normal P-wave does not exceed 0.12sec and its height does not exceed 2.5mm

- The P-waves should be upright in I, II, and V2 to V6

- The first part of the P-wave comes from the right atrium and the second part from the left atrium

The P-wave can be thought to have two components. The first half of the P-wave is made mainly by the right atrium. The second half comes from the left atrium. The best two leads to examine the P-wave are leads II and V1 as they look at the atria in opposite directions. These two leads are typically used as rhythm strips as they emphasis the P-wave. (Lead II looks along the axis of the atria, and V1 looks across the atria.) Disease processes that cause strain on the right atrium cause a typical enlargement of the first half of the P-wave. This gives a taller, peaked P-wave. Lung disease could lead to right atrial strain and thus this tall P-wave is known as P pulmonale. Enlargement of the left atrium causes exaggeration of second part of the P-wave. This leads to the typical bifid "m" shape in lead II, and larger negative deflection in second part of the P-wave in lead V1. This is called P mitrale. (See figure 4.)

59

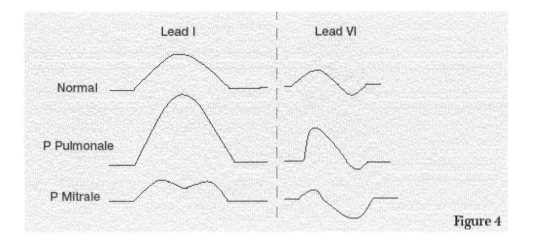

Figure 4

The PR interval

The PR interval starts from the beginning of the P-wave (SA node depolarisation), and includes the whole P-wave--that is, the whole of atrial depolarisation. There is then a flat segment as depolarisation reaches the AV node and there is an electrical interlude. The AV node delays conduction of the electrical impulse long enough so that the ventricles are filled by atrial contraction before they themselves contract. The PR interval ends as ventricular depolarisation begins (the start of the QRS complex). Thus disease of the sinus node, atrial tissues, or AV node could affect the formation and passage of electricity prior to ventricular contraction, and can thus be seen as affecting the PR interval.

Key facts about PR interval

- Represents the time it takes for the atria to depolarise and pass its message to the ventricles

- Is a function of the SA node, atrial tissue and AV node

- Is measured from the beginning of the P-wave to the beginning of the QRS complex (a better description would be PQ interval, but that would perhaps make medicine too easy to understand)

- PR interval should be 0.12 to 0.21 sec (or three to five little squares)

- Prolonged in heart block (discussed later)

- Shortened in conditions where there is an abnormality in the fibrous insulating ring such that the electrical message gets past the AV node quicker--for example, Wolf-Parkinson-White (WPW) and Lown-Ganong-Levine syndromes (discussed later).

QRS-wave

After traversing the AV node, the impulse reaches the Bundle of His and thus it's right and left bundle branches which rapidly conduct it to the ventricular myocardium through the Purkinje fibres. (See figure 5.)

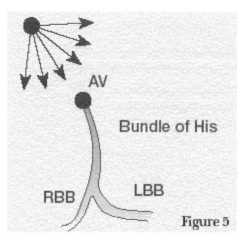

Figure 5

The QRS complex represents ventricular contraction. Were the ventricles to be the same size as the atria and without a specialised path of conduction then the QRS complex would look similar to a P-wave. However because their size and relative bulk is much greater, a specialised conduction system is required to ensure the ventricular muscle all contracts in a synchronous, rapid, and efficient manner. It is in fact quite remarkable that the whole of activation of the ventricle is so rapid, being as quick as the much smaller atria. This rapid activation of such a bulk of muscle creates a large spiked complex. A typical QRS complex is shown in figure 1. Remember, as with the P-wave the complex looks different depending on where it is being recorded from. (See figure 6.)

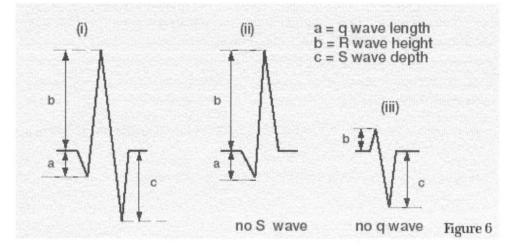

Figure 6

QRS complexes are not always so narrow. We will look at this again when we discuss right and left bundle branch blocks, pacemaker complexes, and broad complex tachycardias. This may sound ominous at the moment but you will be able to work out yourself very simply what you would expect to see in an ECG tracing in these different situations.

Key facts about QRS complex

- Spread of depolarisation from the AV node to all parts of the ventricles takes 0.08-0.1 sec

- If QRS width is >0.12sec (three small squares) it suggests a defect in the conduction system

- No precordial Q-wave must be greater or equal to 0.04 sec (one small square)

- Precordial Q-waves must not have a depth greater than a quarter of the height of the R-wave in the same lead

- The R-wave in the precordial leads must grow from V1 to at least V4

- There should be no Q-wave or only a small q less than 0.04 seconds in width in I, II, V2 to V6

There is a fair amount of muscle in the interventricular septum. This is, of course, the first bit of the ventricle to be depolarised. Activation actually starts at the left side of the interventricular septum and crosses to the right. The wave of depolarisation then spreads down the septum to the apex of the heart. It returns along the outer ventricular walls towards the AV groove. The initial movement is from left to right across the septum. We have already said that speed and mass of the left ventricular activation predominates the major deflection seen in the QRS complex. The mean QRS "axis" describes the average direction of the various electrical forces that develop during ventricular activation, and is of course impelled by left ventricular energy. This axis is described in the standard vertical plane. Similar to the direction shown for the P-wave in figure 2, figure 8 illustrates that the normal average direction of the QRS lies between aVL (-30^0) and aVF (+120^0). Thus lead II will have a large positive QRS. Lead aVR will see the wave going directly away from it--a maximal negative deflection. aVL is perpendicular to this wave front and thus has a smaller biphasic QRS.

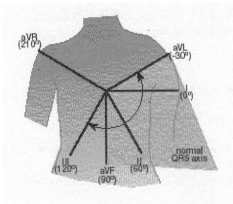

Figure 8

Lastly, Q-waves in the wrong place can be a sign of previous myocardial damage--for example, after a myocardial infarction. However, as we have seen you would normally expect to see an initial negative deflection in certain leads. Where this deflection is greater than that outlined above, the Q-waves are defined as pathological--meaning suggestive of a disease process.

T-waves
This wave represents repolarisation of the ventricles. The returning to normal of the ventricle after depolarisation. (Note: the wave that would represent atrial repolarisation occurs during the QRS complex and is therefore not seen.) It is normally positive in I, II, V4-6 (see figure 9). The T- wave and the ST segment are the most sensitive areas of the ECG in terms of looking at disease processes affecting the ventricle. Unfortunately, the changes are not always specific to a single disease. But there are certain patterns which we can recognise. There is no strict criteria for the size of the T-wave. Generally the tallest precordial T-waves are found in V3 or V4 and the smallest in V1 and V2. As a general rule the T-wave should not be less than one eighth and not more than two thirds of the height of the preceding

R- wave in each of the leads V3-6. It is peaked in hyperkalaemia (high potassium) and flattened in hypokalaemia (low potassium).

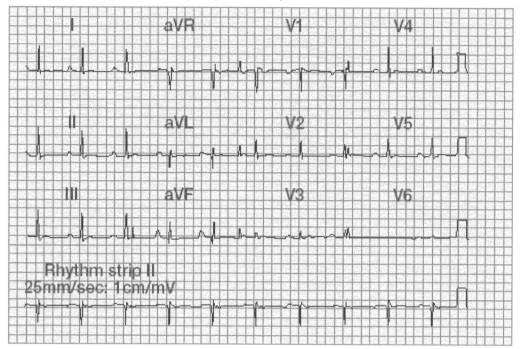

The ST segment

The ST segment lies between the QRS and the T-wave. The normal ST segments do not deviate above or below the isoelectric line (see figure 1) by more than 1 mm. Again we will return to this later as this is one of the disease sensitive areas of the ECG.

Key facts about ST segments

- Elevation of >1mm implies infarction

- Depression of >0.5mm implies ischaemia--for example, angina

- Widespread saddleshaped elevation occurs in pericarditis

QT interval

This is measured from the start of the QRS to the end of the T-wave. The length of this varies with rate. Prolongation of this parameter can be an inherited condition --for example, Romano-Ward and Jervell-Lange-Nielsen syndromes--or acquired--for example, secondary to drugs, toxins, and electrolyte disturbances. These conditions are rare but their significance is that they predispose such patients to potentially serious ventricular arrhythmias. We should emphasise that these conditions are rare and a description is included in this article only for completeness.

The information we have discussed in this article is a mixture of some things you just have to remember such as the names of the waves on the ECG, and some things you have to understand, such as the way in which electricity moves in the heart and creates either an upward or downward deflection on the ECG. A little time spent understanding these concepts is the key to understanding the whole ECG. The ECG in the disease state does become a matter of pattern recognition.

Tachycardias

Tachycardias are the most exciting part of learning about ECGs. It is of course important to understand the mechanism causing tachycardias, but it is equally important to remember to look at the patient first. "Benign" arrhythmias can compromise a person, and "serious" arrhythmias can be asymptomatic. Look at the patient and act with commonsense, rather than treating the ECG.

We are not going to try to explain the emergency treatment of arrhythmias, but this should be something on all doctors' minds (and hearts). All the emergency treatment protocols are available from the European Resuscitation Council (website www.erc.edu/).

Tachyarrhythmias can be divided into two broad categories: supraventricular tachycardias (SVT) and ventricular tachycardias (VT). It is useful to think of these as narrow complex (QRS complex <120ms) tachycardias (SVT) and broad complex (QRS >120 ms) tachycardias (VT).

Why is the QRS complex narrow?

As described above, normally the atrium passes the sinoatrial (SA) node's signal to the atrioventricular (AV) node. This then passes on through the ventricular specialised conducting tissue, which gives rapid, synchronous activation of the whole of the ventricle. Thus to get a narrow complex you must have an electrical signal that passes forward through the AV node, and you must have specialised conducting tissue, that works. A broad QRS complex means that either your conducting system is not working (bundle branch block) or the electrical circuit is not involving the AV node correctly.

So what causes arrhythmias?

Only two things cause abnormal heart rhythms. The most common mechanism involves an abnormal electrical circuit which allows the heart beat to cycle around it. This is called re-entry. The other is where a focal area of the heart starts to "spark off" and send out a shower of extra heart beats (increased automaticity or triggered activity; see figure 1).

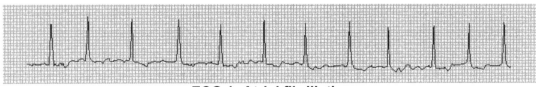
ECG 1: Atrial fibrillation

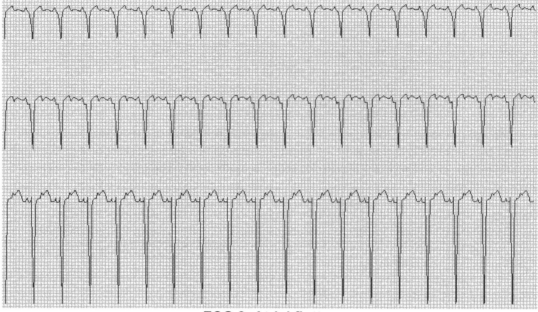

ECG 2: Atrial flutter

Narrow complex tachycardias

Atrial fibrillation (AF)

- The most common sustained arrhythmia of all

- Affects 2% of 65-75 year-olds, 5% over 75 years

- Associated with any disease affecting the heart

- Other narrow complex tachycardias can degenerate to AF--for example, atrial flutter

- Re-entrant mechanism.

Arrhythmia anatomy: Multiple wavelets of re-entry swashing around the atria. The AV node is inundated with cascades of chaotic activity (see figure 2).

ECG: Irregular ventricular rate with no true P waves, baseline irregularities representing atrial activation (ECG 1).

Useful drugs: anticoagulation to prevent thromboembolism; ß blockers, sotalol, propafenone, flecainide, and amiodarone to prevent paroxysmal AF; digoxin ß blocker, diltiazem, and verapamil (often in selected combinations) to control heart rate.

Atrial flutter

- Mistakenly thought of as a variant of atrial fibrillation

- Occurs at any age

- Can be difficult to control with drug therapy

- Re-entrant mechanism.

Arrhythmia anatomy: Typically involves a large circuit created by the structures in the right atrium (figure 3).

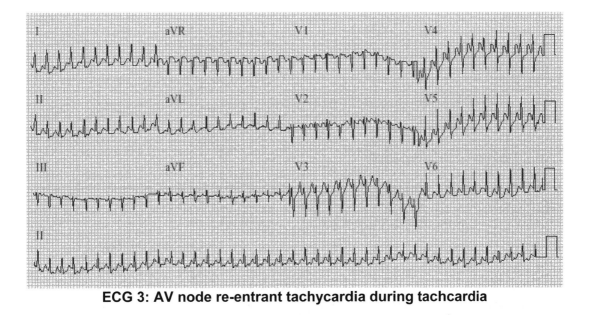

ECG 3: AV node re-entrant tachycardia during tachcardia

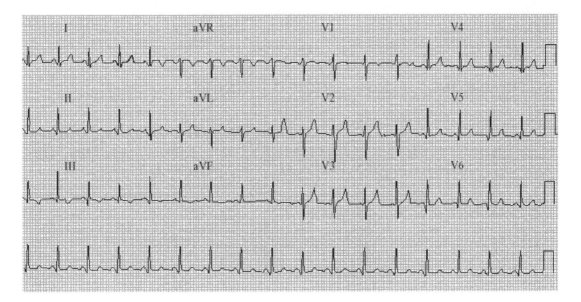

ECG 4: The same patient with AV node re-entrant tachycardia now in sinus rhythm. The QRS complex in lead V1 no longer has a second small R wave, which was due to backward atrial depolarisation occurring at the same time as the QRS during palpitations

ECG: Saw tooth baseline with atrial rate of 300 and ventricular response of 150. Always be suspicious of flutter if you see a narrow QRS tachycardia at a heart rate of 150(ECG 2). Flutter waves are seen before each QRS and after each QRS in the middle of each T wave.

Useful drugs: Digoxin and verapamil (or diltiazem) can be used to slow the response of the AV node. You still get an atrial rate of 300 but hopefully a slower ventricular rate. Type 1c agents (propafenone or flecainide) can be used to stop the atrial circuit and terminate the tachycardia.

Atrioventricular nodal re-entry tachycardia (AVNRT)

- Also known as AV nodal tachycardia (AVNT), or AV junctional tachycardia (AVJRT)

- Commonest type of narrow QRS

- Typically starts in the later teens and 20s

- Re-entrant mechanism.

Arrhythmia anatomy: The basis of this arrhythmia is that the AV node can have two pathways as part of it (see figure 3). These paths allow a circuit to be set up at the AV node itself, giving rise to the arrhythmia.

ECG: Narrow QRS tachycardia of about 180 bpm with P waves often absent: they are hidden in the QRS, as atrial and ventricular depolarisation occur at the same time. You may see changes in the QRS complex in lead V1 as compared with the resting ECG: these are due to simultaneous P wave activation. This is a small positive deflection before the onset of the T wave and is shown in ECG 3 and 4. Look at the subtle difference in the QRS during tachycardia and during normal rhythm.

Useful drugs: Drugs which affect the AV node--that is, digoxin, diltiazem, and verapamil; adenosine can acutely stop the tachycardia as it transiently blocks the AV node (as can vagotonic manoeuvres); ß blockers; type 1c agents (propafenone or flecainide).

Atrial tachycardias

- Second most common SVT

- Can occur at any age, but increased likelihood if the atria are diseased (hypertension, pulmonary disease, previous cardiac surgery, etc)

- Either focal automatic activity (mainly) or due to re-entrant mechanism. Can have multiple foci of automatic activity.

Arrhythmia anatomy: Varied anatomical basis (see figure 4): they can be due to a focal area in the atria with increased automaticity, or re-entry around an abnormal area of atrial tissue.

ECG: Abnormal looking P waves; may have different types of P waves on same ECG. Heart rate very variable from 140 to 240 bpm.

Useful drugs: ß blockers; verapamil or diltiazem; type 1c agents (propafenone or flecainide); amiodarone.

Atrioventricular re-entrant tachycardia (AVRT) and Wolff-Parkinson-White syndrome

- Can occur from infancy onwards

- In infants it may be associated with congenital heart defects

- Re-entrant mechanism

- One to three people in every 1000 have an obvious extra pathway on the resting ECG--that is, Wolff Parkinson White syndrome. It may even be you!

Arrhythmia anatomy: The re-entry mechanism is due to a congenital addition of a small piece of atrial tissue which crosses the isolating fibrous ring separating the atria and ventricles. This gives a large circuit with the heart beat passing down through the AV node, around the ventricle, back up the pathway, and across the atrium back to the AV node. This illustrates why SVT is not such a good name for these arrhythmias: most of this tachycardia's circuit lies in the ventricle.

ECG: The resting ECG can be normal but it can show evidence of the pathway's existence if the path allows some of the atrial depolarisation to pass quickly to the ventricle before it gets though the AV node (Wolff-Parkinson-White (WPW) syndrome; ECG 5). The early depolarisation of part of the ventricle leads to a shortened PR interval and a slurred start to the QRS (delta wave). The QRS is narrow; the message via the AV node eventually predominates because it uses the rapid conducting system to depolarise most of the ventricle.

The tachycardia ECG may be unremarkable, with P waves absent (hidden in the QRS). If the circuit is long or slow enough the P wave may occur at the end of the QRS and can be visible as a distortion in the T wave (this is best seen in lead V1).

Useful drugs: ß blockers; adenosine can acutely stop the tachcardia as it transiently blocks the AV node (as can vagotonic manoeuvres); type 1c agents (oropafenone or flecainide); type 1a agents (procainamide or quinidine).

Atrial fibrillation has an atrial rate of 300-600 bpm. Fortunately, the AV node protects the ventricle from experiencing such a heart rate. In patients with accessory paths there is a mechanism for this very fast heart rate to bypass the AV node and cause AF with a dangerously fast ventricular response (ECG 1). Treating this with drugs such as digoxin, verapamil, or diltiazem would further block the AV node but not prevent the AF from passing down the accessory path. The situation would be made a lot worse in this case. This is why the drugs are stated as being contraindicated in atrial fibrillation in the presence of an accessory pathway.

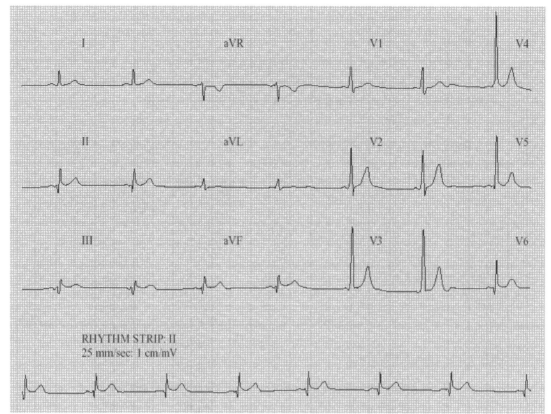

ECG 5: Wolff-Parkinson-White syndrome

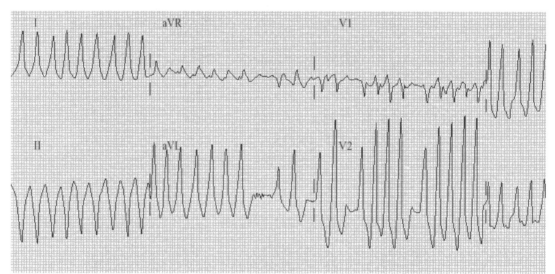

ECG 6: A patient with AF and an accessory pathway. The ECG is irregular and frighteningly quick (more than 300bpm in places)

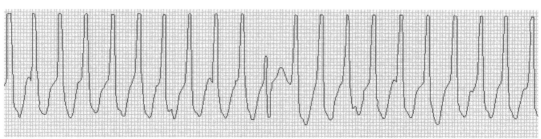

ECG 7: Ventricular tachycardia: AV dissociation

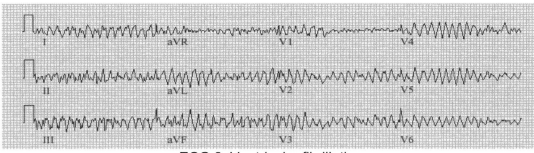
ECG 8: Ventricular fibrillation

Broad complex tachycardias

To have a narrow complex you need functioning specialised conducting tissue, and the cardiac impulse must pass through the AV node normally. All of the SVTs can give a broad complex tachycardia if bundle branch block is present. Much time is spent by cardiologists considering ECGs and asking whether they show VT or SVT with bundle branch block. To the majority of doctors it does not matter. Think of it as VT and you will do little harm in the acute situation. Always treat the patient and not the ECG. So if you see a broad complex tachycardia look at the patient.

Ventricular tachycardia

- Broad complex tachycardia means ventricular tachycardia until proved otherwise

- Likely in patients with established heart disease

- Mainly, but not exclusively, re-entrant mechanism (see figure 6).

ECG: Broad complex >120 ms; bizarre QRS morphology; no P waves preceding each QRS; abnormal axis; concordant QRS (all point in the same direction); capture or fusion beats may be present (see ECG 7).

Useful treatments: Check the patient; if the patient is pulseless get help and treat as per resuscitation guidelines.

Ventricular fibrillation (VF)

- VF is the rapid, totally uncoordinated contraction of ventricular myocardial fibres

- Causes circulatory arrest; unconciousness develops within 10 to 20 seconds.

ECG: Irregular, chaotic electrical activity (ECG 8).

Useful treatment: Defibrillation.

The main message about tachycardias is at all times to assess the patient, not treat the ECG. Obviously, ventricular arrhythmias cause most concern as they are most likely to upset the heart's ability to pump blood effectively. But remember that relatively benign rhythms can be devastating if they are fast enough or in a patient with little physiological reserve. If the patient is well there will be enough time to assess even the most serious rhythm disturbance. If the patient is threatened by their heart rhythm then following life support protocols is essential. These give everyone dealing with the situation a proper structure so that they can think and act together.

Bradycardias

Symptoms from slowing of the heart can be very varied, from sudden death, recurrent syncope, and epileptic-type fits, to much milder symptoms, such as lethargy, breathlessness, etc. The history can be very revealing, but can also be very unreliable in those patients who truly lose consciousness. Some bradycardias are only intermittent problems with bothersome recurrent blackouts but no abnormality found after many years of medical investigation. Getting evidence of an intermittent problem can be very difficult.

Bradycardia is "slow" cardiac rhythm and results from either a failure of initiation of the heart beat or failure of passage of this electrical message through the heart--that is, normal sinus node "spark plug" activity is disturbed or there is interruption of the passage of this activity to tell the pump to work. This second type of failure usually occurs at the atrioventricular (AV) node.

The intrinsic rate of the sinoatrial (SA) node, which controls the heart rate in normal circumstances, is 60 to 70 beats per minute, and a bradycardia is defined as a pulse rate of <60 beats per minute. Such a rate may be physiological (and therefore acceptable) in athletes, young people, or during sleep, but it can be of profound clinical significance resulting from acute myocardial infarction, sick sinus syndrome, or from a variety of different drugs--for example, beta blockers. Several non-cardiac disorders, such as hypothyroidism, hypothermia, jaundice, and raised intracranial pressure can also cause sinus bradycardia.

Identifying the important different types of bradycardias is relatively straightforward and will be considered in turn: sick sinus syndrome (sinoatrial disease); carotid sinus hypersensitivity; vasovagal syndrome; AV heart block; agonal rhythm; asystole.

Likewise the treatment options are few in number and basically consist of removing or treating the underlying cause: (a) resuscitation with drugs to stop the heart slowing (atropine); (b) drugs to speed up the heart (isoprenaline); (c) pacing the heart electrically.

The first three conditions are predominantly problems with the SA node or its innervation.

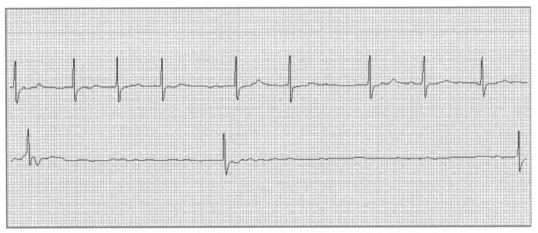

ECG 1: Patient who has gone into slow atrial fibrillation

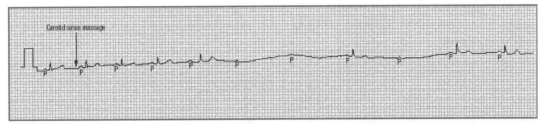

ECG 2: This ECG of a young patient undergoing cartoid sinus massage shows profound slowing of the P wave rate. There is lengthening of the PR interval and then complete loss of ventricular activity for over 3 and a half seconds

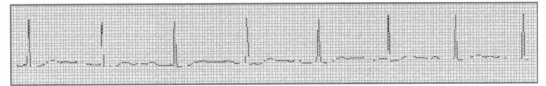

ECG 3: First degree heart block: a constant prolonged PR interval

Sick sinus syndrome (SSS)

This is common in the elderly and is usually caused by idiopathic degeneration of the SA nodal cells. Sinoatrial disease may be associated with coronary artery disease, particularly that involving the right coronary artery, although many of these patients have normal coronary arteries. It causes bradycardia that can be profound enough to cause arrest; SA block; or supraventricular tachycardia (SVT) alternating with bradycardia ("tachy-brady syndrome").

Patients may be completely asymptomatic, in which case usually no treatment is indicated. They can present with symptomatic bradycardia, dizziness, or syncope. The diagnosis is from 12 lead or 24 hour ambulatory ECG recording and, importantly, demonstrating a correlation between periods of bradycardia, or sinus pauses, and symptoms. It is accepted that a pause of over three seconds is significant. (ECG 1)

Normal PR interval (because this is an SA node, not an AV node, problem). Every P wave is followed by a normal QRS complex (unless dual pathology), but there are periods when interval between P waves (P-P interval) is prolonged.

Treatment: Removal of extrinsic causes of bradycardia and/or permanent pacemaker (PPM) implantation. Note that in the tachy-brady syndrome once a PPM has been implanted medications which would normally slow the intrinsic cardiac rate can then be used to control the SVT--for example, beta blockers.

Carotid sinus hypersensitivity

Similar symptoms to SSS can occur due to a hypersensitive carotid sinus reflex. It is diagnosed by finding either a sinus pause or of AV block greater than three seconds in response to five seconds of carotid sinus massage. Again where an association is made between symptoms and ECG findings then PPM is indicated.

Note that carotid sinus massage affects both SA and AV nodes, therefore as well as a sinus bradycardia the PR interval can also be prolonged resulting in AV block [ECG2]

Vasovagal syndrome

This is a common condition, particularly in younger people, and a more malignant variety is recognised in the more elderly. This vagally mediated bradycardia can be treated by PPM.

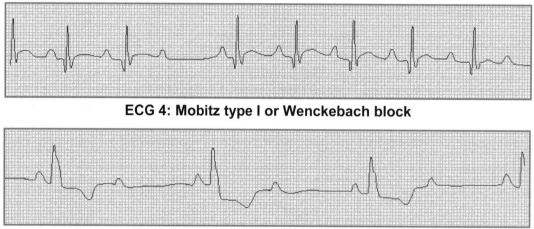

ECG 4: Mobitz type I or Wenckebach block

ECG 5: Mobitz type II second degree atrioventricular (2:1)

AV heart block

AV heart block is divided into first, second, and third degree AV blocks, which as the names suggest, involve a problem at the AV node!

All three variants involve the association between the P wave and the QRS complex. Because the problem is not with the SA node or the ventricular polarisation itself, then both the P wave and QRS complex commonly look normal. It is the association between the two that is seen to be different, and this is because they are connected via the AV node. Causes of AV block are shown in the box.

Causes of AV block

- Acute myocardial infarction or ischaemia

- Drugs--beta blockers, verapamil, digoxin, Class I antiarrhythmics

- Infection--diphtheria, rheumatic fever, endocarditis, Lyme disease

- Idiopathic fibrosis of the conducting system

- Infiltration--sarcoidosis, syphilis, scleroderma, tumour, calcific aortic stenosis

First degree AV block

The PR interval is prolonged (>0.20 sec) but constant (ECG3).This does not produce any symptoms and does not require any active treatment.

Second degree AV block

There are two types of second degree block:

Möbitz type I (also known as Wenckebach) has a progressively lengthening PR interval that eventually drops a QRS complex and starts over with a progressively lengthening PR interval before dropping a QRS complex again (ECG 4). This is normally associated with a reliable subsidiary pacemaker and a lower chance of progressing third degree block. Pacemaker implantation is not mandatory without evidence of correlated symptoms or undue bradycardia.

Möbitz type II is different in that the PR interval is constant but occasionally a P wave is not conducted through the AV node and is therefore not followed by a QRS complex--that is, there is a "dropped beat." Regular non-conducted P waves may result in a high degree block. If only every second or third P wave is followed by a QRS complex then there is said to be 2:1 block or 3:1 block respectively. (ECG 5) Type II AV block usually indicates an extensive infranodal abnormality and therefore, except in the context of an acutely reversible condition, requires a permanent pacemaker.

Third degree AV block (complete heart block)

In this, there is regular firing of the SA node giving regular P waves. The P waves, however, do not get through the "broken" AV node. Most cardiac tissue can produce some spontaneous activity. The lonely ventricle now electrically separated from the atrium usually produces its own slow heart rhythm. Often this comes from near the start of the His Purkinje system, leading to a narrow normal complex QRS. If the complex arises more distally then the complex cannot be propagated in the normal manner. It therefore takes longer to transmit across the ventricle and therefore the QRS complex looks wider. (ECG 6) A permanent pacemaker is essential, even if asymptomatic, as there is a risk of sudden death.

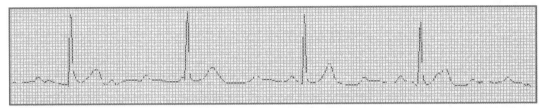

ECG 6: Third degree or complete heart block. There is clearly no association between the frequent P waves and narrow complex ventricular rhythm.

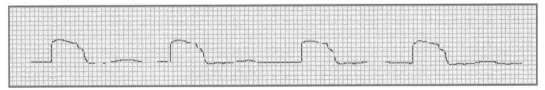

ECG 7: Agonal rhythm

Agonal rhythm

This is a slow, irregular rhythm with wide ventricular complexes of varying morphology, which is often seen during the later stages of unsuccessful resuscitation attempts as the heart dies. The complexes become progressively broader before all recognisable activity is lost. (ECG 7)

Pacemakers

Pacemakers treat all types of bradycardia and also interfere with and abort many tachycardias. They can also be used to re-coordinate ventricular function in patients with heart failure and damaged electrical conducting systems. Most pacemakers listen to the heart's own rhythm and leave things alone as long as things are working properly. If the heart beat changes they then step in to stimulate the heart appropriately.

To do this the pacemaker is comprised of three parts: the wires, the battery, and the computing system. Most wires or leads are placed inside the heart via the subclavian or other vein. Sometimes leads are placed on the surface of the heart (epicardial) via opening the chest in a more invasive procedure. These wires are the permanent part of the system. The battery and computer are inside a can which attaches to the leads.

Asystole

This is not really a bradycardia, rather a complete cessation of both atrial and ventricular activity. If the ECG shows asystole and the patient is speaking to you then you need to check that your leads are properly attached. If there are persisting P waves but no ventricular activity then it is called ventricular standstill.

The emergency treatment of most bradycardias is atropine, a pacemaker, or sympathomimetic drugs, such as adrenaline or isoprenaline. The need for treatment depends on the haemodynamic consequences of the arrhythmia, which is not likely to be significant unless the rate drops below 40 beats per minute.

Bradycardia can occur just because someone is fit; many professional athletes will have a heart rate around 40 beats per minute. Bradycardia is also a major cause of blackouts, and can be very difficult to diagnose if it occurs rarely and is intermittent. Patients who black out will not always be aware of truly losing consciousness and may even "remember" tripping over.

Understanding ECGs adapted/reproduced from

sBMJ 2001;09:357-398 October, sBMJ 2001;09:399-442 November,sBMJ 2001;09:443-486 December

with permission from the BMJ Publishing Group.

ECG in Bundle Branch Block

"WiLLiaM MoRRoW":
W pattern in V1-V2 and **M** pattern in V3-V6 is **L**eft bundle block.
M pattern in V1-V2 and **W** in V3-V6 is **R**ight bundle block.
· Note: consider bundle branch blocks when QRS complex is wide.

Causes of ST elevation

ELEVATION:
Electrolytes
LBBB
Early repolarization
Ventricular hypertrophy
Aneurysm
Treatment (eg pericardiocentesis)
Injury (AMI, contusion)
Osborne waves (hypothermia)
Non-occlusive vasospasm

DEPRESSED ST:
Drooping valve (MVP)
Enlargement of LV with strain
Potassium loss (hypokalemia)
Reciprocal ST- depression (in I/W AMI)
Embolism in lungs (pulmonary embolism)
Subendocardial ischemia
Subendocardial infarct
Encephalon haemorrhage (intracranial haemorrhage)
Dilated cardiomyopathy
Shock
Toxicity of digitalis, quinidine

Causes of T-wave inversion

INVERT
Ischemia
Normality [esp. young, black]
Ventricular hypertrophy
Ectopic foci [eg calcified plaques]
RBBB, LBBB
Treatments [digoxin]

The Respiratory System

General Respiratory History

		Not attempted	Attempted inadequate	Attempted adequate
1	Approaches the patient politely and introduces him/herself.	0	1	2
2	Asks the patient's name, DOB and occupation.	0	1	2
3	Asks about history of cough.	0	1	2
4	Asks about history of shortness of breath.	0	1	2
5	Asks about history of chest pain.	0	1	2
6	Asks about history of wheeze.	0	1	2
7	Asks whether the patient has noticed any recent weight loss.	0	1	2
8	Asks about the occurrence of fever or night sweats.	0	1	2
9	Asks about relevant past or current conditions including TB, pneumonia, DVT / PE, asthma and chronic bronchitis or emphysema.	0	1	2
10	Asks about family history of respiratory disease particularly TB, cystic fibrosis and emphysema.	0	1	2
11	Asks a detailed occupational history.	0	1	2
12	Asks about smoking and alcohol consumption.	0	1	2
13	Asks about home circumstances including pets.	0	1	2
14	Asks about past and current medications and any allergies to medication.	0	1	2

1. It is polite and professional to introduce yourself.
2. Name: to establish rapport and identify the patient.
   Age/DOB: certain diseases affect certain age groups, e.g. lung carcinoma is rare in the young. The DOB should be recorded to identify the patient.
   Occupation: this can give useful background information about the patient. It is also particularly relevant for respiratory disease as many conditions have links to occupational exposure.
3. See specific history for cough.
4. See specific history for dyspnoea.
5. Chest pain due to respiratory disease is usually sharp and exacerbated by deep inspiration or coughing. It is commonly localised to one area of the chest.
   Pleuritic pain is often associated with dyspnoea and may be due to pneumonia, pulmonary embolus or pneumothorax.
   Localised anterior chest pain accompanied by costochondral junction tenderness is suggestive of costochondritis.
   Pain in the shoulder tip indicates irritation of the diaphragmatic pleura.

6. Wheeze is caused by airflow limitation, which can be due to asthma, chronic airways disease or a foreign body or tumour. It is usually expiratory; inspiratory wheeze (stridor) suggests large airways obstruction.
7. Weight loss may be a marker of malignancy but also occurs in severe chronic airflow limitation due to the increased respiratory effort required.
8. Fever can be a symptom of a respiratory infection. Night sweats are characteristic of TB, pneumonia and lymphoma, amongst others.
9. A history of previous respiratory infections predisposes to further episodes. Increased breathlessness, sputum volume and purulence characterise exacerbations of underlying chronic disease.
    Patients with repeated DVT / PE should be investigated for thrombophilia.
    TB has many extra pulmonary manifestations, which can occur years after the original infection. Reactivation of the pulmonary infection can also occur, often in the presence of diabetes mellitus, malnutrition, immunosuppression, HIV infection or drugs.
10. TB can be spread to close contacts so all close family members should be screened.
    Cystic fibrosis is an inherited disease.
    Alpha-1 antitrypsin deficiency is an inherited condition, which predisposes to the development of emphysema.
11. Ask the patient to describe in detail what their occupation involves and which dusts, fumes or vapours they are exposed to. In particular, a history of exposure to asbestos should be sought.
    It is important to find out whether they are provided with protective clothing or masks and whether any other workers have become ill.
    Exposure to mouldy hay, humidifiers or air conditioners can result in allergic alveolitis. A history of working with animals, including birds is also relevant.
    An improvement of symptoms over weekends or holiday periods when the patient is not at work is strongly suggestive of an occupational cause.
12. Smoking is the major cause of chronic airflow limitation and lung cancer.
    Passive smoking is also a risk so exposure at home or work should be asked about.
    Alcoholics are at risk of aspiration pneumonia.
13. The impact of symptoms needs to be considered in relation to the patient's lifestyle e.g. the levels of disability that breathlessness causes depends on the activities that the patient is used to carrying out.
    Pet antigens can cause asthma.
    Bird keeping is a risk factor for extrinsic allergic alveolitis and psittacosis.
14. Chronic respiratory diseases may have been treated with steroids and these can predispose to reactivation of TB.
    Many classes of drug can produce respiratory side effects e.g. cough from ACE inhibitors, interstitial lung disease from methotrexate or cyclophosphamide and bronchospasm from β-blockers or NSAIDs.
    Some non-prescription drugs e.g. cocaine can also cause lung disease.
    Intravenous drug users are at risk of lung abscesses and drug-related pulmonary oedema.

Presenting Complaint - Cough

		Not attempted	Attempted inadequate	Attempted adequate
1	Asks the patient how long they have had a cough.	0	1	2
2	If chronic, asks whether the cough has changed in character recently.	0	1	2
3	Asks if the cough is dry or productive.	0	1	2
4	Asks how much sputum the patient produces per day.	0	1	2
5	Asks about consistency, colour and odour of the sputum.	0	1	2
6	Asks whether the patient has ever coughed up blood.	0	1	2
7	Asks at which time of day their cough is worst and whether it keeps them awake at night.	0	1	2
8	Asks the patient whether their cough is made worse by particular conditions such as pollen, dust or cold air.	0	1	2
9	Asks the patient if they have an associated wheeze, chest pain or shortness of breath.	0	1	2
10	Asks about the occurrence of fever / night sweats.	0	1	2
11	Asks if the patient feels systemically unwell.	0	1	2
12	Asks if the patient has noticed any weight loss.	0	1	2
13	Asks the patient if they suffer from indigestion or acid regurgitation.	0	1	2
14	Asks if they have travelled abroad recently or been in contact with anyone with pneumonia.	0	1	2
15	Asks if the patient has a history of asthma, COPD or TB.	0	1	2
16	Asks if they use inhalers or any other medications.	0	1	2
17	Asks if they work in a dusty environment.	0	1	2
18	Asks if they smoke.	0	1	2
19	Asks about history of childhood respiratory disease.	0	1	2
20	Asks if they have had a BCG immunisation.	0	1	2

1. A cough of recent onset is most likely to be due to an infective cause, especially if other signs such as a fever are present.
   A chronic cough can be due to a number of conditions including asthma, COPD, GOR or the use of ACE inhibitors.

2. A change in character of a chronic cough may indicate a new underlying problem such as an infection or malignancy.

3. In bronchiectasis and chronic bronchitis, the cough is productive whereas ACE inhibitors and GOR typically cause a dry cough.

4. Large volumes of sputum are produced in bronchiectasis.
A patient with COPD will produce more sputum than is usual for them during an infective exacerbation.

5. Bronchiectasis and lobar pneumonia lead to purulent, yellow / green sputum being produced.
If there is a lung abscess, the sputum is often darker and foul smelling.
Sputum produced in asthma is usually yellow.
Pink frothy sputum is produced in pulmonary oedema.

6. Haemoptysis should be regarded as suspicious of lung cancer until proved otherwise. Other causes include TB, bronchiectasis, pulmonary infarction, trauma, generalised bleeding disorders and arteriovenous malformations.

7. The coughs of asthma and heart failure are typically worse at night whereas 'smokers' coughs' are worse in the morning. A cough that is worse following eating or drinking suggests GOR.
Whether the cough keeps the patient awake at night gives an indication of its severity and how much disruption it is causing. A psychogenic cough will disappear during sleep.

8. These are recognised trigger factors for allergic reactions and suggest that asthma should be considered as the cause of the cough.

9. Cough, wheeze, pleuritic chest pain and shortness of breath can occur together in asthma, COPD and chest infections.

10. See point 7 of the general respiratory history.

11. Systemic upset suggests that an infectious cause should be sought.

12. Weight loss may be indicative of malignancy.

13. GOR may be associated with cough.

14. A history of recent travel should alert you to consider infectious diseases that are common in the area visited. TB is present world-wide but is particularly prevalent in Asia and Africa.
Pneumonia in a patient who has been abroad needs to be treated with antibiotics which will cover atypical organisms.

15. Patients with COPD are prone to chest infections.
Cough can be a sign of poorly controlled asthma.
TB in an adult may be the result of reactivation of old disease.

16. Both COPD and asthma are usually managed with inhaled drugs. Find out which inhalers the patient has been prescribed and how often they use them.
ACE inhibitors can cause a dry cough.

17. See point 11 of the general respiratory history.

18. Smoking is a major risk factor for lung disease.

19. Pneumonia and whooping cough in childhood may give rise to bronchiectasis in adulthood.
Childhood asthma may re-present later in life with a cough.
Progressive cough and sputum from childhood raises the possibility of cystic fibrosis.

20. BCG vaccine is offered to neonates considered to be high risk and then to children requiring it following the Mantoux test at age 10-13. It is effective for approximately 10 years in up to 80% of subjects.

Presenting Complaint - Shortness Of Breath

(This symptom may also be a feature of cardiovascular disease)

		Not attempted	Attempted inadequate	Attempted adequate
1	Asks the patient to describe the sensation they experience.	0	1	2
2	Asks how long ago they first noticed feeling breathless.	0	1	2
3	Asks if they have any chest pain.	0	1	2
4	Asks if the breathlessness is constant or if it comes and goes.	0	1	2
5	Asks what activities the patient is unable to do because of the breathlessness and how far they can walk on flat ground.	0	1	2
6	Asks whether the level of exertion at which the patient gets short of breath is increasing or staying the same.	0	1	2
7	Asks whether anything makes the breathlessness better or worse.	0	1	2
8	Asks whether the patient can lie flat without becoming breathless and how many pillows they have to use at night.	0	1	2
9	Asks whether the patient ever wakes up breathless from sleep.	0	1	2
10	Asks whether they have noticed swelling of their legs or ankles.	0	1	2
11	Asks whether there is associated wheeze, cough or systemic illness.	0	1	2
12	Asks whether they have a history of asthma, COPD or cardiac disease.	0	1	2
13	Asks whether the patient smokes.	0	1	2
14	Asks whether the patient uses inhalers.	0	1	2
15	Asks whether they ever get tingling in their fingers or feel light-headed when they are short of breath.	0	1	2

1. People describe many different sensations as 'breathlessness'. They may be describing a feeling of being tight chested, unable to get their breath, unable to fill the bottom of their lungs or functional disability such as being unable to do the vacuuming.

2. Sudden dyspnoea can be due to an inhaled foreign body, pneumothorax, PE or asthma.
   Dyspnoea developing over a few hours is more likely to be due to asthma, pneumonia, pulmonary oedema or extrinsic allergic alveolitis.
   Dyspnoea developing over a few days suggests asthma, pleural effusion or pulmonary oedema.
   Dyspnoea over months or years is suggestive COPD, fibrosing alveolitis or non-respiratory causes such as anaemia.

Malignancy usually causes breathlessness over a period of weeks, but the onset may be rapid depending on the exact position of the lesion.

3. MI, pneumothorax and PE can all cause chest pain and breathlessness.

4. Variable, intermittent dyspnoea may be due to asthma or pulmonary oedema.

5. This tells you about the impact of the symptom on the patient's life as well as being a guide to the severity of the dyspnoea. Asking about specific circumstances such as climbing stairs or walking on the flat can be useful.

6. This tells you whether the underlying cause is static or progressive.

7. Triggers such as dusting, exercise and cold air exacerbate asthma.

8. Patients with breathlessness due to heart disease characteristically experience it on lying flat (orthopnoea). However, this is also a feature of severe fixed airways obstruction.
   The number of pillows patients prop themselves up with to sleep is a guide to the severity of the condition.

9. Paroxysmal nocturnal dyspnoea characteristically occurs in patients with pulmonary oedema from left ventricular failure, where it is often accompanied by a cough with pink frothy sputum. However, asthmatics may develop bronchoconstriction in the night and wake with wheeze and breathlessness.

10. Ankle oedema is a feature of right sided (or congestive) heart failure. It can also occur due to stasis in elderly patients.
    Unilateral calf swelling may be a sign of a DVT and should alert you to the possibility of a PE as the cause of the shortness of breath.

11. Wheeze in association with shortness of breath points to small airway obstruction.
    Cough can be a feature of poorly controlled asthma or of respiratory infection. Systemic illness, such as pyrexia, myalgia and headache, suggests the cause may be infective.

12. Shortness of breath can be the presenting feature of an exacerbation of asthma, COPD or cardiac failure.

13. Smoking is a major risk factor for respiratory and cardiovascular disease.

14. This tells you that they have a history of respiratory disease.
    Find out what inhalers they use and how often they need them.

15. These symptoms can be caused by the reduction in pCO_2 that occurs with hyperventilation.

Examination of the Respiratory System

		Not attempted	Attempted inadequate	Attempted adequate
1	Approaches the patient politely and introduces him/herself. Exposes the patient adequately after obtaining their permission	0	1	2
2	Performs a general inspection of the patient and their surrounds from the end of the bed.	0	1	2
3	Feels for the rate and regularity of the radial pulse whilst recording the respiratory rate and commenting on cachexia, dyspnoea, stridor and use of accessory muscles of respiration.	0	1	2
4	Inspects the hands and nails commenting on clubbing, palmar erythema, peripheral cyanosis, wasting of the small muscles of the hand, coal dust tattoos and nicotine stains.	0	1	2
5	Tests for the flap of CO_2 retention.	0	1	2
6	Inspects the conjunctivae for pallor and comments on any constriction of the pupils or ptosis.	0	1	2
7	Looks at the tongue for central cyanosis.	0	1	2
8	Looks for a raised JVP.	0	1	2
9	Looks for tracheal tug and feels for deviation of the trachea after warning the patient that it may be uncomfortable. If it is deviated, feels to see if the apex beat is also displaced.	0	1	2
10	Inspects the chest, commenting on scars, shape and movement with respiration.	0	1	2
11	Assesses degree of chest wall expansion by palpation.	0	1	2
12	Assesses tactile vocal fremitus.	0	1	2
13	Percusses the chest wall mapping out any areas of altered resonance.	0	1	2
14	Auscultates the lungs commenting on the character and intensity of the breath sounds and the presence or absence of any added sounds.	0	1	2
15	Assesses the character of vocal resonance.	0	1	2
16	Asks the patient to sit forward and repeats inspection, palpation, percussion and auscultation over the back.	0	1	2
17	Palpates cervical and scalene lymph nodes.	0	1	2
18	Feels the sacrum and ankles for oedema.			
19	Thanks patient and washes hands	0	1	2

1. It is important to introduce yourself and explain that you would like to examine their chest. Explain that you need to expose them fully in order to perform an adequate examination but always respect the modesty of patients. Explain what you are going to do as you proceed with the examination, *before* you do it!
2. Assess whether the patient looks comfortable at rest or unwell.
   Important clues around the bedside include oxygen, sputum pots and inhalers.
3. Tachycardia is a feature of severe asthma or infection.
   The normal respiratory rate at rest should be less than 15 breaths / minute. It is increased in fever and severe lung disease.
   Cachexia is a feature of malignancy and TB.
   Stridor is inspiratory noise caused by large airway obstruction.
   Use of accessory muscles implies increased work of breathing.
4. Respiratory causes of clubbing include lung cancer, fibrosing alveolitis, lung abscess, bronchiectasis and empyema.
   Wasting of the small muscles of the hand can be caused by lung cancer involving the brachial plexus.
   Peripheral cyanosis in the absence of central cyanosis is due to reduced / slow peripheral circulation (in which case the peripheries will be cold).
   Red, warm, clammy palms may indicate CO_2 retention.
5. Ask the patient to hold their arms out with their wrists dorsiflexed and their fingers apart. Severe CO_2 retention leads to a flapping tremor but this is a late sign.
6. Pale conjunctivae are a sign of anaemia.
   Apical lung cancer can compress the sympathetic nerves in the neck, causing Horner's syndrome with ipsilateral constriction of the pupil and partial ptosis.
7. The underside of the tongue is the best place to observe central cyanosis. It is a late sign of hypoxaemia.
8. A raised JVP is suggestive of right heart failure, which may be secondary to chronic lung disease (cor pulmonale).
9. In severe airflow obstruction, the trachea descends on inspiration (a tracheal tug). Feel for tracheal deviation by placing three fingers in the jugular notch. The trachea deviates towards the pathological side in fibrosis or simple pneumothorax. It deviates away from the pathological side in tension pneumothorax or massive pleural effusion.
   An associated displaced apex beat suggests lower mediastinal shift.
10. The anteroposterior diameter increases in emphysema (barrel shaped chest).
    Pectus carinatum (pigeon chest) can be from childhood asthma or rickets (or can be a developmental abnormality).
    Pectus excavatum (funnel chest) is usually congenital and asymptomatic.
    Kyphosis and scoliosis can restrict lung movement.
    Inspection of chest wall movement can be used to gain a crude idea of degree of movement and any asymmetry.
    Scars caused by operative procedures or radiotherapy are important clues to the underlying pathology.
11. This is done by placing your fingers as far round the back of the chest as possible with your thumbs in the midline and lifted slightly off the chest so that they are free to move. Thumb movement can then be used as a measure of chest expansion.
    <5cm is generally pathological. <2cm is definitely pathological.
    Asymmetrical expansion indicates abnormal underlying lung (pleural effusion, pneumothorax, consolidation or fibrosis). Reduced expansion bilaterally indicates a diffuse abnormality such as chronic airways disease or fibrosing alveolitis.

12. Place the ulnar borders of your hands on the chest wall and compare the vibrations on either side asking the patient to say 'ninety nine'. Repeat the procedure at three positions down the chest.
    Vibrations will be transmitted more readily and felt more strongly over consolidated lung. They will be absent over an area of collapse, pleural effusion or pneumothorax (see vocal resonance below).
13. Percuss symmetrical areas of chest wall covering each zone and comparing equivalent levels on both sides.
    The sound is characteristically stony dull in pleural effusion, dull in fibrosis, consolidation or collapse and hyperresonant in emphysema and pneumothorax.
14. Auscultate at three positions over the chest wall, comparing sides.
    The sounds of normal air entry are known as vesicular.
    Bronchial breath sounds are loud inspiratory and expiratory blowing sounds which are associated with lung consolidation or pulmonary fibrosis.
    Wheezes are musical sounds on exhalation produced by turbulent flow in narrowed airways.
    Early inspiratory crackles may indicate obstruction in the central airways. Late inspiratory crackles are a sign of shrunk lungs (fibrosing alveolitis, pneumonia, heart failure) and are posturally dependent (normally heard at the bases). They can be cleared by deep coughs if due to excess secretions.
    A pleural rub is the creaking sound of inflamed pareital over visceral pleura. It remains unchanged after coughing and is often associated with localised pain.
15. Vocal resonance is assessed by asking the patient to say 'ninety nine' whilst you auscultate, again comparing sides.
    Lung consolidation leads to increased vocal resonance so whispering is clearly audible (whispering pectoriloquy). The sound is decreased if there is air, fluid or pleural thickening between the lung and the chest wall.
16. Percuss and auscultate round to the mid-axillary line. Asking the patient to bring his / her elbows together in front of the chest moves the scapulae out of the way and makes examination easier.
17. These are enlarged in respiratory infection, malignant infiltration, sarcoidosis and HIV infection. Palpation should be done with the patient sitting forwards and you standing behind them.
    Start under chin and feel for submental nodes in the midline.
    Work back feeling for sub-lingual, sub-mandibular and then tonsillar nodes.
    Feel for the jugular digastric node at the top of the anterior chain.
    Work down the anterior chain (in front of sternomastoid) and back up the posterior chain (behind sternomastoid).
    Feel behind the mastoid processes for the pre-auricular nodes.
    Move round to the back of head to feel for sub-occipital nodes.
    Feel for supra- and infra-clavicular nodes.
18. Ankle oedema occurs in cor pulmonale.
19. It is polite to thank the patient. Always wash your hands to reduce the risk of cross-infection.

	Consolidation	Pleural effusion	Lobar collapse	Pneumothorax	Pleural thickening
Chest xray					
Mediastinal shift	No	No or away	Towards	No (simple), away (tension)	No
Chest wall excursion	Normal or decreased	Decreased	Decreased	Normal or decreased	Decreased
Percussion note	Normal or decreased	Decreased (stony)	Decreased	Increased	Decreased
Breath sounds	Increased (bronchial)	Decreased	Decreased	Decreased	Decreased
Added sounds	Crackles	Rub (occassional)	None	Click (occassional)	None
Tactile vocal fremitus/vocal resonance	Increased	Decreased	Decreased	Decreased	Decreased

Reproduced from sBMJ 1997:February:9-10 with permission from the BMJ Publishing Group.

88

Top Tips

Looking at Chest X-Rays

You will need to develop a system for looking at x-ray films. This will reduce your chances of missing abnormalities and it will provide a structured description to come out with, especially in exams when you are under pressure.

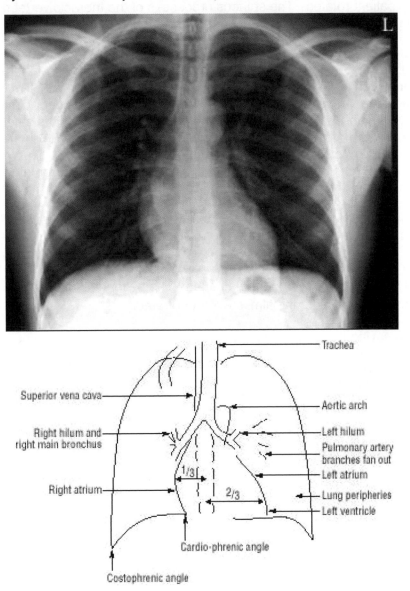

Fig 1: Normal Chest X-Ray

Let's start by looking at a normal chest x-ray film (fig 1). Use this film as a reference point during the rest of this part. Firstly, some technical details: Quickly look at the film to get some useful information about the patient:

- Male or female? Look for the presence of breast shadows (this will help you to notice a mastectomy too).

- Old or young? Try to use the patient's age to your advantage by making sensible suggestions. A 20 year old is much less likely to have malignancy than someone who is 70.

- Good inspiration? It's easy to get tied up in knots over this - and sometimes not get any further. The diaphragms should lie at the level of the sixth ribs anteriorly. The right hemidiaphragm is usually higher than the left because the liver pushes it up.

- Good penetration? You should just be able to see the lower thoracic vertebral bodies through the heart.

- Is the patient rotated? The spinous processes of the thoracic vertebrae should be midway between the medial ends of the clavicles.

- Most chest x-ray films are taken posterior anterior (PA) - that is, the x-rays shoot through from the back of the patient to the x-ray plate in front of the patient. If the patient is too sick to stand up for this, an anterior posterior (AP) film will be done - that is, the x-rays shoot through from front to back. An anterior posterior film will always be labelled as AP, so if nothing is written on the film it is safe to assume it is PA. PA films are better, particularly because the heart is not as magnified as on an AP film, making it easier to comment on the heart size. Tip: You can avoid the whole PA/AP debate by describing all chest x-ray films "frontal" - that is, you are looking at the patient straight on.

- Finally, some examiners like you to call x-ray films radiographs; strictly speaking you can't actually see the x-rays themselves.

You can summarise all the above information in a simple opening phrase: "This is a frontal chest radiograph of a young male patient. The patient has taken a good inspiration and is not rotated; the film is well penetrated."

While you are saying this keep looking at the film.

- First look at the mediastinal contours - run your eye down the left side of the patient and then up the right.

- The trachea should be central. The aortic arch is the first structure on the left, followed by the left pulmonary artery; notice how you can trace the pulmonary artery branches fanning out through the lung (see fig 1).

- Two thirds of the heart lies on the left side of the chest, with one third on the right. The heart should take up no more than half of the thoracic cavity. The left border of the heart is made up by the left atrium and left ventricle.

- The right border is made up by the right atrium alone (the right ventricle sits anteriorly and therefore does not have a border on the PA chest x-ray film - a question that examiners love to ask. Above the right heart border lies the edge of the superior vena cava.

- The pulmonary arteries and main bronchi arise at the left and right hila. Enlarged lymph nodes can also occur here, as can primary tumours. These make the hilum seem bulky - note the normal size of the hila on this film.

- Now look at the lungs. Apart from the pulmonary vessels (arteries and veins), they should be black (because they are full of air). Scan both lungs, starting at the apices and working down, comparing left with right at the same level, just as you would when listening to the chest with your stethoscope. The lungs extend behind the heart, so look here too. Force your eye to look at the periphery of the lungs - you should not see many lung markings here; if you do then there may be disease of the air spaces or interstitium. Don't forget to look for a pneumothorax - in which case you would see the sharp line of the edge of the lung.

- Make sure you can see the surface of the hemidiaphragms curving downwards, and that the costophrenic and cardiophrenic angles are not blunted - suggesting an effusion. Check there is no free air under the hemidiaphragm.

- Finally look at the soft tissues and bones. Are both breast shadows present? Is there a rib fracture? This would make you look even harder for a pneumothorax. Are the bones destroyed or sclerotic? (see fig 2)

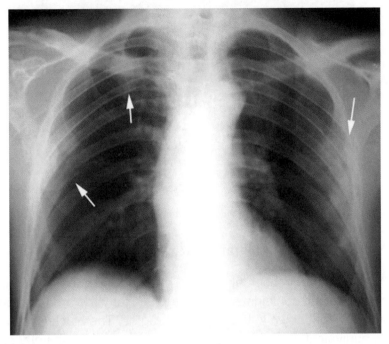

Fig 2: Sclerotic-white metastasis

You can summarise your findings as you are looking: "The trachea is central, the mediastinum is not displaced. The mediastinal contours and hila seem normal. The lungs seem clear, with no pneumothorax. There is no free air under the diaphragm. The bones and soft tissues seem normal."

If you have not seen any abnormality by this point, say so - "I have not yet identified an abnormality so I will now look through my review areas" - and then look at the "review areas" - places where you can easily miss disease. These are: apices, periphery of the lungs, under and behind the hemidiaphragms (don't forget the lungs will extend here), and behind the heart. By the time you have gone through the above, showing that you are looking at the film in a logical fashion, the examiner should guide you towards the abnormality.

You may be shown a lateral chest x-ray (see fig 3), usually to confirm a diagnosis you have made on the PA film. Therefore don't panic when the lateral goes up because it means you've probably made the diagnosis. There are only two spaces to look at on the lateral film.

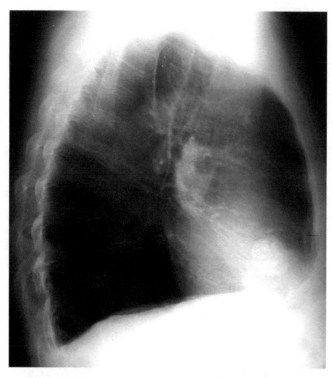

Fig 3: Lateral chest *x-ray* (normal)

The heart lies antero-inferiorly. Look at the area anterior and superior to the heart. This should be black, because it contains aerated lung. Similarly the area posterior to the heart should be black right down to the hemidiaphragms. The blackness in these two areas should be equivalent; therefore you can compare one with the other. If the area anterior and superior to the heart is opacified, suspect disease in the anterior mediastinum or upper lobes. If the area posterior to the heart is opacified suspect collapse or consolidation in the lower lobes.

The trachea and mediastinum are deviated

The trachea can be pulled or pushed, almost always by one of three processes (two that push, one that pulls). A right sided pleural effusion will push the trachea and mediastinum to the left (fig 4). Similarly, a left sided tension pneumothorax will push the mediastinum to the right, as air builds up in the left pleural space and cannot be released (fig 5).

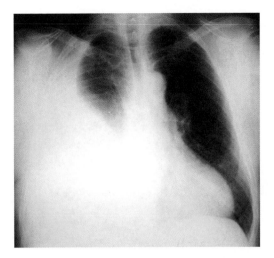

Fig 4: Right-sided pleural effusion pushing mediastinum to the left

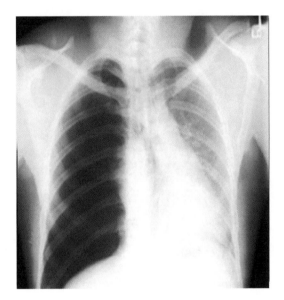

Fig 5: Right tension pneumothorax pushing mediastinum to the left

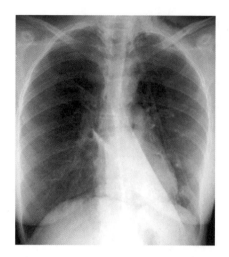

Fig 6: Left lower lobe collapse with shift of the mediastinum to the left

On the other hand, if there is collapse on the left this will pull the trachea and mediastinum to the left side (fig 6). Most other processes (consolidation, nontension pneumothorax, etc) have little effect on the mediastinum. If you see the mediastinum is shifted then you need to think of these three things and look for them.

An enlarged heart

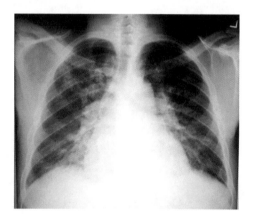

Fig 7: Left Ventricular Failure

The most common reason for the heart to be enlarged is congestive cardiac failure, so look for signs of left ventricular failure on the rest of the film (fig 7). These are:

1. Upper lobe blood diversion. The pulmonary veins running from the upper lobes seem more prominent than those running from the lower lobes.

2. Kerley B lines. These are tiny horizontal lines from the pleural edge and are typical of fluid overload with fluid collecting in the interstitial space.

3. "Bat's wing" haziness around the hila.

4. Alveolar shadowing. In very severe pulmonary oedema fluid collects not only in the interstitial space but in the air spaces or alveoli. You can recognise this by seeing hazy shadowing throughout the lungs, and possibly air bronchograms.

There are only a few occasions when there may be the appearance of left ventricular failure (LVF) but a normal sized heart - in an acute myocardial infarct (sudden onset of LVF), or lymphangitis carcinomatosa may mimic the appearances of LVF and be accompanied by a normal sized heart.

Enlarged hila

This could be due to an abnormality in any of the three structures which lie at the hilum.

- The pulmonary artery - for example, pulmonary artery hypertension, secondary to mitral valve disease; chronic pulmonary emboli; or primary pulmonary hypertension (fig 8).

- The main bronchus - carcinoma arising in the proximal bronchus (fig 9).

- Enlarged lymph nodes - caused by infection, such as tuberculosis - spread from a primary lung tumour; lymphoma; or sarcoidosis (fig 10).

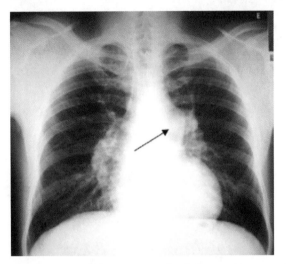

Fig 8: Primary pulmonary hypertension, both right and especially left pulmonary arteries are enlarged

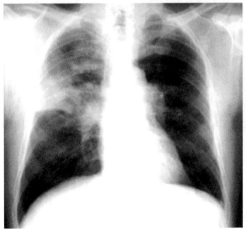

Fig 9: Right hilar carcinoma

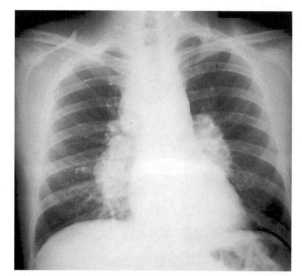

Fig 10: Bilateral hilar lymphadenopathy due to sarcoidosis

Pneumothorax

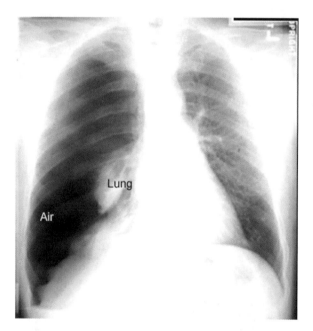

Fig 11: Right pneumothorax. The right side of the lung is blacker, and the lung edge is seen. There is no mediastinal shift and therefore no tension

It is important to view around the periphery of the lungs to look for a pneumothorax (air in the pleural space with associated collapsed lung). It is very easy to miss a pneumothorax. Watch out for the following signs:

- One half of the lung may seem blacker - that is, more radiolucent - than the other, which will be more radio-opaque or whiter. In particular, the area beyond the collapsed lung will be very radiolucent because there are no pulmonary vessel markings.

- You should be able to identify the edge of the collapsed lung (see fig 11).

Having identified a pneumothorax you need to look for several more associated abnormalities:

- Most importantly - this is a pass or fail observation - is there evidence of a tension pneumothorax? This occurs when air can enter the pleural space (via a hole in the lung surface or the chest wall) but, because of a ball-valve effect, air cannot leave by the same route. So more and more air accumulates in the pleural space. This pushes the mediastinum over to the opposite (normal) side and eventually compresses the normal lung so that less inspiration occurs on the normal side, with compression on the heart and decreased venous return until finally the patient arrests (see fig 12). Always look for this and say: "There is no shift of the mediastinum and therefore no tension pneumothorax" or "There is shift of the mediastinum away from the side of the pneumothorax indicating a (right/left) tension pneumothorax. This is a medical emergency which I would treat immediately by inserting a large bore cannula into the (right/left) pleural space."

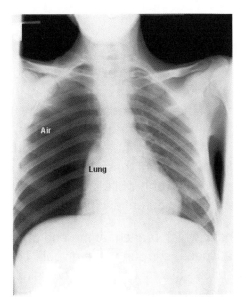

Fig 12: Right tension pneumothorax with shift of the mediastinum to the left.

- The cause of the pneumothorax may be apparent - for example, fracture of the ribs.

- There may be associated surgical emphysema - that is, air in the soft tissues - and air in the mediastinum (see fig 13).

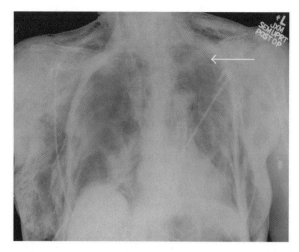

Fig 13: Surgical emphysema (outside chest) and pneumomediastinum

There is extra shadowing in the lungs

It may be difficult to work out what is causing extra shadowing in the lungs, especially near the mediastinum where normal structures may overlay the extra shadowing. It is useful to look at the periphery of the lungs because normally the outermost edge of the lungs should be fairly black with a few tapering blood vessels. If you do see more shadowing in the periphery then there may be either **interstitial or air space disease**. As examiners often show films with one of these two types of shadowing, understanding the difference between these two is worth while because it will help you to interpret what you see and lead you to the correct differential diagnosis.

The lung is made up of bronchi, which branch, at the end of which are alveoli. The interstitial space (or potential space) surrounds the alveoli. The whole of the lung from bronchi to alveoli is the air space - that is, it normally contains air. But the air spaces can fill up - with **fluid** (such as in severe pulmonary oedema), with **pus** (as in infection), with **blood** (as in rare diseases such as Goodpasture's syndrome, associated with renal failure), or with **tumour cells** (alveolar carcinoma).

Fluid and pus are more common than the second two. When the air spaces fill up, the alveoli fill first, with the bronchi being relatively spared. Therefore the bronchi, which are still air filled, stand out against the alveoli, which are filled with pus or fluid. This is called an air bronchogram and is simply a sign that there is air space disease. Consolidation is another term for air space shadowing (see figs 14 and 15). If there is air space disease then you need to work out which part of the lungs it is affecting. A quick way is to use the word "zone" to describe which part of the lung is affected. Say something like "There is shadowing in the air spaces of the right mid and lower zone." You can then take your time to work out which lobe is affected. You can find out more about lobar anatomy in the later section on collapse and consolidation.

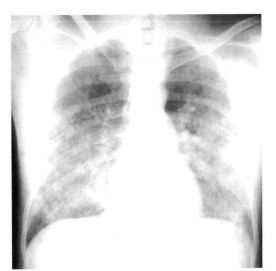

Fig 14: Left and right lower lobe air space shadowing in an ITU patient

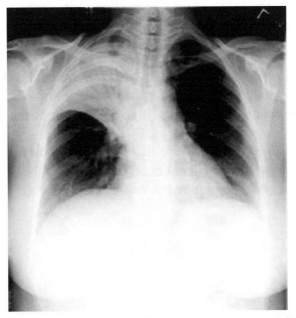

Fig 15: Right upper lobe consolidation/air space shadowing. Note air bronchogram . There is no loss of volume, which is a key feature of consolidation

Let's turn to the interstitial space. This surrounds bronchi, vessels, and groups of alveoli. When there is disease in the interstitium it manifests itself by **reticulonodular shadowing** (criss cross lines or tiny nodules or both). The main two processes affecting the interstitium are **accumulation of fluid** (occurring in pulmonary oedema or in lymphangitis carci- nomatosa) and **inflammation leading to fibrosis** (occurring in industrial lung dis- ease, inflammatory arthritides such as rheumatoid arthritis, inflammation of unknown cause such as cryptogenic fibrosing alveolitis and sarcoidosis). If you see criss cross lines or tiny nodules or both say: "There is reticulo-nodular shadowing within the lower zones." (See figure 16.)

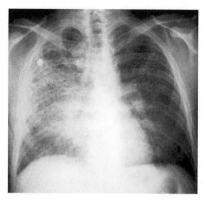

Fig 16: Recticular-nodular shadowing caused by lung fibrosis (circled). Note how the heart has lost its normal smooth outline and seems "shaggy"

Abnormality: lobar collapse

Collapse of a lobe is caused by proximal Obstruction - for example, by a neoplasm, mucus plug, such as in a postoperative patient, or foreign body, such as in a child. Always mention that you are looking for the cause of the collapse.

When the lobe is not aerated it will lose much of its volume and collapse to a predictable location depending on whether it is an upper, middle, or lower lobe. Figure 17 shows the normal site of the lobes of the lung; figures 18 to 24 and their accompanying line diagrams show where the lobes collapse to. The collapsed lobe itself can be very difficult to see - there may simply be a little extra shadowing on the film. A collapsed lobe is a cause of volume loss; the other cause is a pneumothorax. The signs that should alert you to a collapse are due to the loss of lung volume:

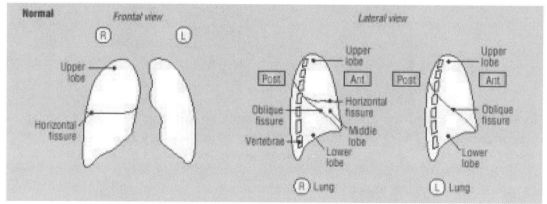

Fig 17: Where the lobes of the lung normally lie

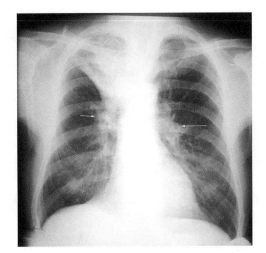

Fig 18: Right upper lobe collapse. Increased shadowing in the right upper zone with a clear linear border of the horizontal fissure which has been pulled up. Note the remaining right lung is blacker than the opposite side. In addition the hilum is pulled up. There is a mass arising from the right hilum; this is the obstructing bronchial carcinoma which is causing the collapse

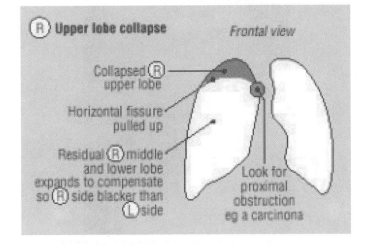

Fig 19: Right upper lobe collapse

- The mediastinum may be shifted towards the side of collapse

- The hilum is pulled up or down from where it normally lies

- The horizontal fissure will also be pulled up (in a right upper lobe collapse) or down (right lower lobe collapse)

- The remaining (non-collapsed) lung on the side of the collapse has to expand to fill the hemithorax, thus "spreading" its contained vessels; therefore the abnormal side will seem blacker with fewer lung markings than the opposite normal side

- The proximal obstruction may be visible - for example, a large carcinoma arising from the right upper lobe.

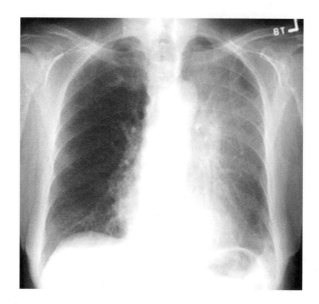

Fig 20: Antero-posterior chest radiograph, left upper lobe collapse

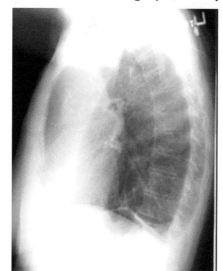

Fig 21: Lateral. Left upper lobe collapse. Increased shadowing in the left upper and mid zone with a blurred lower border. The left heart border is also lost, because the lung collapses adjacent to it. On the lateral view the upper lobe can be seen to have collapsed anteriorly and lies anterior to the oblique fissure

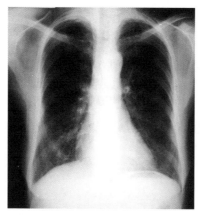

Fig 22: Antero-posterior chest radiograph. Right middle lobe collapse. The right middle lobe lies adjacent to the right heart border, so the right heart outline is lost.

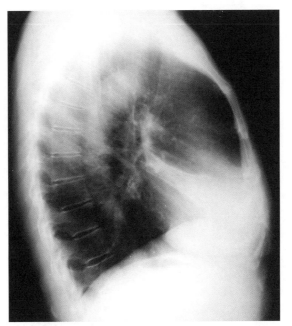

Fig 23: Lateral, same patient. The right middle lobe collapses anteriorly in a wedge shape over the heart. The upper border of the wedge is the horizontal fissure, the lower border is the oblique fissure

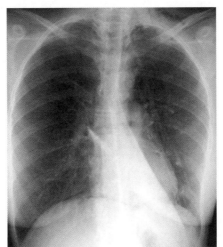

Fig 24: Antero-posterior chest radiograph. Left lower lobe collapse. The lower lobes collapse posteriorly and inferiorly so that the contour of the hemidiaphragm is lost. The collapsed left lower lobe may form a "sail" shape behind the heart border on the Antero-posterior film

Abnormality: confluent opacification of the hemithorax

There are four main causes of confluent opacification of a hemithorax - **consolidation** (fig 27) (that is, material within the air-spaces) and **pleural effusion** - that is, material within the pleural space, which could be serous fluid, blood, or pus (fig 29). **Complete collapse of one lung** with the mediastinum shifting over the the abnormal side can also cause a "white out" on the abnormal side (fig 30). Finally, after a **pneumonectomy** the mediastinum shifts to the empty hemithorax and the residual pleural space fills with fluid and fibrotic material leaving the patient with a complete "white out" on the side that has been operated on (fig 31). Consolidation and pleural effusion are the two most common, and it can be difficult to distinguish between them - of course, they can coexist.

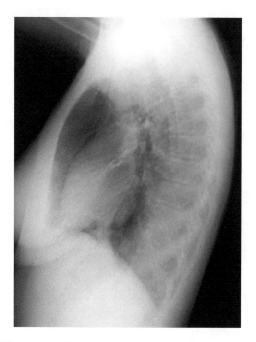

Fig 25: On the lateral film there is extra shadowing posteriorly over the vertebrae due to the collapsed lobe

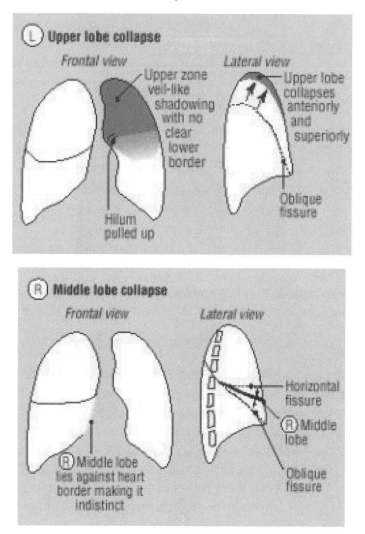

104

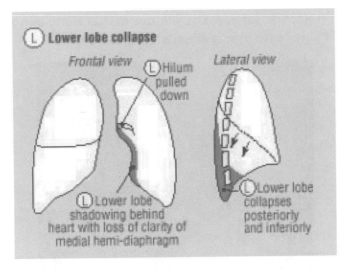

Fig 26: Left upper, middle and lower lobe collapse

Effusion

The key features of an effusion are:

- If the patient is erect there should be a fluid level and meniscus visible

- If the effusion is large the mediastinum will be shifted to the opposite side. Compare this with pure consolidation in which there is no change in volume of the hemithorax and therefore no mediastinal shift. There is one caveat to bear in mind, which is that if collapse of the lung is accompanied by a pleural effusion the loss of volume (caused by the collapse) may be balanced out by the increase in volume of the hemithorax (caused by the effusion) and therefore it may seem as if the volume of the hemithorax overall is equivalent to the opposite side.

The key feature of consolidation is an air bronchogram. In infective causes of consolidation the process may affect a lobe (lobar pneumonia in a distribution according the normal anatomy shown in fig 17) or spread in a more patchy distribution (bronchopneumonia).

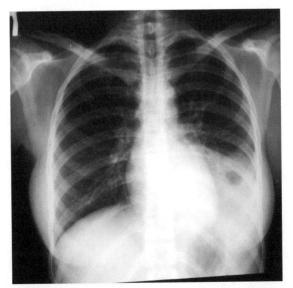

Fig 27: Left lower lobe consolidation. There is opacification of the left lower zone with loss of the hemidiaphragm, indicating the consolidation abuts the diaphragm

- that is, is within the lower lobe. A key feature is that there is no loss of volume. There is no mediastinal shift and no fluid level

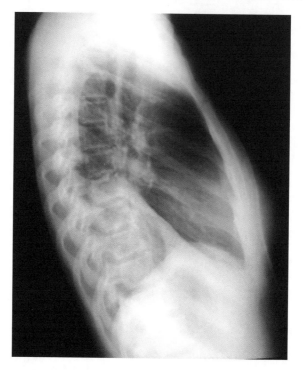

Fig 28: On the lateral film, air bronchograms can be seen within the consolidation which occupies the posterior lower hemithorax-that is, the normal anatomical site of the left lower lobe

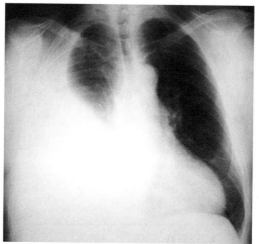

Fig 29: Right pleural effusion. There is opacification of the lower right hemithorax with a fluid level, and the mediastinum is pushed to the left side

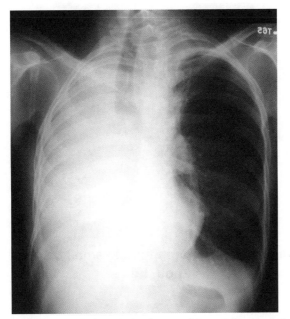

Fig 30: Complete collapse of the right lung. A proximal right main bronchus carcinoma has obstructed the distal right bronchus and caused complete collapse of the right lung with the trachea and mediastinum pulled to the right side by the loss of volume on the right. There is also a right sided pleural effusion, best seen superiorly. However, the loss of volume due to the right lung collapse is greater than the increase in rightsided volume due to the pleural effusion so that overall the mediastinum is pulled over to the right

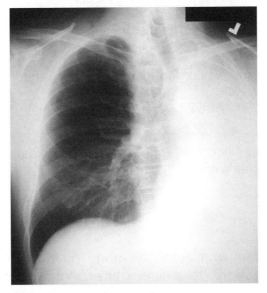

Fig 31: Left pneumonectomy. The left lung contained a carcinoid tumour and was removed. There is left sided loss of volume with shift of the mediastinum and chest wall (ribs) and left hemidiaphragm towards the "empty" left hemithorax. The residual space in the left hemithorax fills with fluid and fibrotic tissue a few weeks after pneumonectomy

Abnormality: multiple discrete nodules in the lungs

Discrete nodules do not have a reticular or linear component. They can be small (up to 5 mm) or large. The differential diagnosis is shown in box 1 and some of them are illustrated in figures 1, 2, and 3.

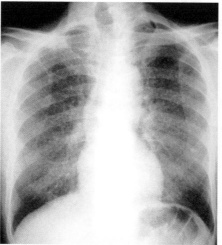

Fig 32: Miliary tuberculosis. There are multiple small discrete nodules throughout both lungs

---

Box 1- Differential diagnosis of small and large lung nodules Small nodules (<5 mm)

- Miliary tuberculosis (so called because they look like tiny seeds "milia"), due to haematogenous spread

- Sarcoid (which can also cause reticulo-nodular shadowing)

- Metastases (although they are usually bigger)

- Pneumoconiosis - for example, due to inhaling coal dust. This is rare nowadays

- Chickenpox pneumonia Larger nodules/masses (>5 mm)

- Common: Metastases (especially breast, testis, gastrointestinal tract, kidney, and thyroid)

- Rare: Inflammatory nodules - for example, due to vasculitis of rheumatoid arthritis or Wegener's granulomatosis

---

Abnormality: single nodule or mass in the lung: The two main causes of a single mass in the lung are: **infection/** - for example, tuberculosis and **neoplasm** - for example, primary bronchial tumour or single metastasis. In both cavitation may occur.

Other causes of single or multiple masses in the lung are rare. Only mention them if pressed by an examiner. They include hydatid cyst and pulmonary arteriovenous malformation.

Tuberculosis (TB)

Turberculosis has various manifestations in the lung. In primary tuberculosis there is a peripheral lung mass (Ghon focus) with enlarged hilar lymph nodes (fig 35).

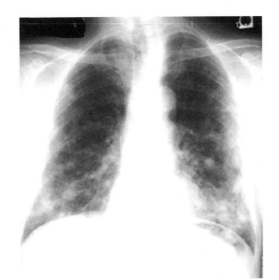

Fig 33: Multiple miliary lung metastases

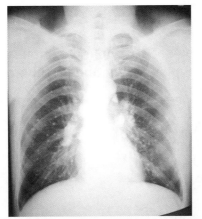

Fig 34: Multiple small calcified lung nodules

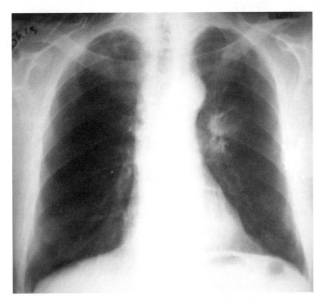

Fig 35: Previous tuberculosis.

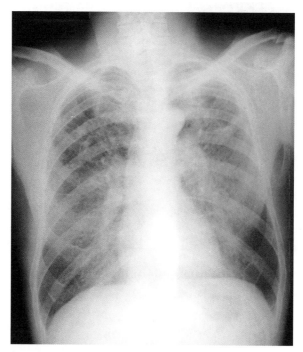

Fig 36: Secondary tuberculosis. Some consolidation in the right upper lobe with a cavity typical of secondary tuberculosis

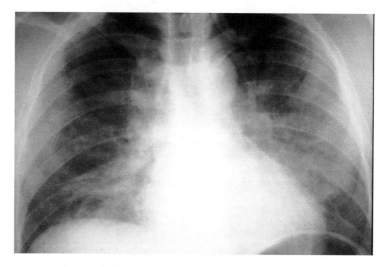

Fig 37: Pneumocystis carinii pneumonia in a patient with AIDs. PCP has varied appearances. Here there is an air space shadowing in the lower zones

Consolidation can also occur. In secondary tuberculosis there is patchy consolidation especially in the upper lobes (fig 36). This can cavitate. Other manifestations include pleural effusions and miliary tuberculosis. Mediastinal lymphadenopathy does not occur in secondary TB. Other infections can cavitate, including pneumonias due to *Staphylococcus*, *Klebsiella,* and *Cryptococcus*. *Pneumocystis carinii*, as the name suggests, can form cysts which are airfilled and have a similar appearance on an x-ray film to cavities (fig 37).

Lung carcinomas can also cavitate, squamous cell carcinomas are the typical histological subtype to do so. Apart from cavitation, other features of lung carcinomas are listed in box 2: they can occur in the periphery of the lung or centrally (in or near the mediastinum). The outline of the tumour may be spiculated. Look for associated pleural effusion or hilar lymphadenopathy.

Proximal tumours can cause distal consolidation or collapse. Local rib destruction or multiple bony metastases can also occur so look for these.

Box 2 - Primary lung carcinoma - features to look for

- Any site (from central to peripheral lung)

- May cavitate

- Spiculated, irregular outline

- Distal consolidation or collapse

- Pleural effusion

- Hilar lymphadenopathy

- Local bony destruction

- Multiple bony metastases

Top-Tips for Chest X-Rays adapted / reproduced from :

sBMJ 2000 September:315-317,sBMJ 2000 October:358-360,sBMJ 2000 November:408-410

sBMJ 2000 December: 444-446,sBMJ 2001 February: 10-12

with permission from the BMJ Publishing Group.

Inhaler Technique

		Not Attempted	Attempted inadequate	Attempted adequate
1.	Introduces self to patient (name and role and purpose of consultation)	0	1	2
2.	Establishes patient's understanding of the treatment	0	1	2
3.	Explains how to use the inhaler correctly • Shake inhaler then remove cap. • Take a deep breath in then fully exhale • seal lips around the mouthpiece • Breathe in through the mouthpiece, while simultaneously pressing down the top of the inhaler. • Continue to breathe in deeply to ensure the medicine gets into the lungs • Hold your breath for 10 seconds or as long as you comfortably can, before breathing out slowly. • If you need to take another puff, wait for 30 seconds, shake your inhaler again then repeat. • Replace the cap on the mouthpiece. • If steroid inhaler – advise use of mouthwash following use	0	1	2
4.	Establishes patient understanding allowing them to demonstrate the technique.	0	1	2
5.	Explains when to take the medication (prophylactic, regular use and acute use)	0	1	2
6.	Clear organised explanation without the use of medical jargon	0	1	2
7.	Invites patient to ask questions	0	1	2
8.	Thanks the patient and washes hands	0	1	2

Peak Flow Measurement

		Not Attempted	Attempted inadequate	Attempted adequate
1.	Introduces self to patient	0	1	2
2.	Explains procedure and obtains verbal consent	0	1	2
3.	Sets peak flow meter to zero	0	1	2
4.	Connects disposable mouthpiece	0	1	2
5.	Asks the patient to stand or if unable, to sit as upright as possible			
6.	Ensures patient's fingers do not obstruct the slide of the peak flow meter	0	1	2
7.	Instructs the patient to inhale deeply, place their lips around the meter, making a tight seal. While holding the meter horizontally, exhale forcefully	0	1	2
8.	Notes the reading	0	1	2
9.	Repeats twice unless the patient is unable to do so	0	1	2
10.	Records the highest of the 3 measurements. If only one reading was able to be taken due to extreme cough / wheeze etc. document that only one reading was taken	0	1	2
11.	Disposes of the mouthpiece and thanks the patient and washes hands	0	1	2

The Neurological System

General Neurological History

		Not attempted	Attempted inadequate	Attempted adequate
1	Approaches the patient politely and introduces him/herself.	0	1	2
2	Asks the patient's name, DOB and occupation.	0	1	2
3	Asks about history of headache and facial pain.	0	1	2
4	Asks about history of neck stiffness.	0	1	2
5	Asks about history of fits or faints.	0	1	2
6	Asks about history of dizziness or vertigo.	0	1	2
7	Asks about disturbances of vision, hearing or smell.	0	1	2
8	Asks whether the patient has any difficulty with walking.	0	1	2
9	Asks about any episodes of sudden onset weakness.	0	1	2
10	Asks about altered sensation in their limbs.	0	1	2
11	Asks about history of disturbances of sphincter control (bladder, bowels).	0	1	2
12	Asks about involuntary movements or tremor.	0	1	2
13	Asks about history of speech and language or swallowing disturbance.	0	1	2
14	Asks about relevant past or current conditions including hypertension, ischaemic heart disease, hypercholesterolaemia, diabetes, stroke, epilepsy, meningitis, head or spinal injuries and previous operations.	0	1	2
15	Asks about risk factors for HIV infection or syphillis.	0	1	2
16	Asks about family history of heart disease, vascular disease and neurological or psychological disease.	0	1	2
17	Asks about smoking and alcohol consumption.	0	1	2
18	Asks about occupational history and exposure to toxins.	0	1	2
19	Asks about home circumstances.	0	1	2
20	Asks about past and current medications and any allergies to medication.	0	1	2

1. It is polite to introduce yourself and explain your task.

2. Name: to establish rapport and identify the patient.
    Age/DOB: certain diseases affect certain age groups, e.g. headache is more likely to have a sinister underlying cause in the very old or very young. The DOB should be recorded to identify the patient.

Occupation: this can give you information about a person's background and can have significant effects on the management of their condition. It is important to determine whether there is the possibility of occupational disease.

3. See specific history for headache and facial pain.

4. Meningism leads to resistance to neck flexion due to painful spasm of the extensor muscles in the neck. It occurs in meningitis and subarachnoid haemorrhage.

5. See specific history for collapse.

6. Dizziness is a word used for a variety of complaints ranging from slight unsteadiness to severe vertigo. It is therefore important to find out in the patient's own words, exactly what they mean by the term.
A sensation of movement of self or surroundings is true vertigo and indicates a disturbance of the vestibular portion of the eighth nerve, brainstem or, rarely, cortical function. It has a number of causes.
Unprovoked attacks of vertigo occur in Meniere's disease (causing the triad of vertigo, tinnitus and deafness) vestibular neuritis and in some ataxic syndromes.

7. Visual problems include decreased acuity, double vision, blurred vision and photophobia.
A loss of the sense of smell is most commonly caused by upper respiratory tract infection but in the absence of this, may be due to a meningioma in the olfactory groove or a basal or frontal skull fracture. Sense of smell is also diminished by smoking and increasing age.
Deafness can be classified into conduction deafness or neural deafness.
Causes of conduction deafness include wax, otitis media, otosclerosis and Paget's disease. Causes of nerve deafness include environmental exposure to noise, tumours, infection, Meniere's disease and drugs eg. aspirin or gentamicin.

8. Gait is best assessed on examination but the patient may describe patterns that they, or others, have noticed.
Common neurological patterns of gait disturbance are described in the examination section.

9. See specific history for sudden onset weakness.

10. Paraesthesiae, numbness and pain are the principal symptoms of lesions of the sensory pathways below the level of the thalamus.
Peripheral mononeuropathies are often due to nerve entrapment eg. carpal tunnel syndrome affecting the median nerve. However, peripheral nerves can also be affected by demyelination, axonal degeneration, infarction or infiltration.
Spinal root lesions lead to tingling discomfort in the dermatome and weakness in the myotome supplied by the root. These are often caused by disc protrusions.
Peripheral polyneuropathies can lead to progressive symmetrical numbness and tingling in the hands and feet, spreading proximally in a glove and stocking distribution. This usually occurs over several months but there are acute and subacute causes such as Guillan-Barre syndrome and vitamin B_{12} deficiency.

11. Neurological causes of incontinence include spinal cord lesions, spina bifida, multiple sclerosis and diabetes mellitus with autonomic involvement.

12. This symptom is best assessed on examination but the patient may describe it. Parkinson's disease characteristically leads to a resting tremor.

Intention tremor is due to cerebellar disease.

An action tremor can be seen in anxiety or thyrotoxicosis or be benign essential tremor.

Chorea consists of involuntary, jerky movements, flitting from one part of the body to the other. Causes include Huntington's disease, Sydenham's chorea (post-infective), drugs (phenytoin, levodopa and alcohol) and thyrotoxicosis.

13. Difficulty with swallowing is most often a symptom of a local oesophageal lesion but can be due to pseudobulbar (bilateral UMN lesions of CN IX, X and XII) and bulbar (bilateral LMN lesions of CN IX, X and XII) palsies.

    Dysarthria (difficulty with articulation) can be caused by lesions of the lower cranial nerves or cerebellum, Parkinson's disease or by local discomfort.

    Dysphasia (language defect) is caused by lesions in the dominant lobe (usually left) and can be classified into receptive, expressive, nominal and conductive.

14. Hypertension, hypercholesterolaemia, diabetes and ischaemic heart disease are all risk factors for cerebrovascular disease.

    Meningitis and head injuries predispose to neurological disease and recurrent headaches.

    Knowledge of previous spinal injuries will identify the likely level of any lesion.

15. These conditions both have neurological complications.

16. A family history of cardiac or vascular disease is a risk factor for the development of similar conditions.

    Some neurological conditions eg. Huntington's, have a genetic predisposition.

17. Smoking predisposes to cerebrovascular disease.

    Alcohol can result in a number of neurological symptoms and conditions including tremor, hallucinations, dementia, peripheral neuropathy, seizures, Wernicke's encephalopathy and Korsakoff's psychosis.

18. Exposure to heavy metals is particularly important to ask about.

    Disorders due to toxins can be of acute onset or develop over months or years.

19. Many neurological disorders are debilitating and patients need considerable physical and psychological support. Patients with neurological symptoms are often very concerned about the underlying cause and likely prognosis.

20. It is important to find out which treatments have been tried already in the case of chronic disorders such as epilepsy and persistent headache.

    Many drugs have toxic effects on the nervous system eg. isoniazid and phenytoin can cause peripheral neuropathies.

    Seizures can be provoked by some medications.

    Anti-epileptic drugs can cause ataxia, diplopia and tremor.

Presenting Complaint - Headache And Facial Pain

		Not attempted	Attempted inadequate	Attempted adequate
1	Asks the patient to indicate where exactly the headache or pain is.	0	1	2
2	Asks the patient to describe the character of the headache or pain.	0	1	2
3	Asks the patient when the headache or pain first began and whether the onset was sudden.	0	1	2
4	Asks if there is anything that makes the headache or pain better or worse and whether the headache or pain is worse at any particular time of day.	0	1	2
5	Asks the patient if the headache or pain is constant or intermittent.	0	1	2
6	Asks the patient to rate the severity of the headache or pain.	0	1	2
7	Asks whether the headache or pain is associated with any visual disturbance.	0	1	2
8	Asks whether the headache or pain is associated with nausea or vomiting.	0	1	2
9	Asks whether there is any associated weakness or sensory disturbance.	0	1	2
10	Asks whether the patient has any other symptoms such as neck stiffness or fever.	0	1	2
11	Asks whether the patient has been under any particular stress recently.	0	1	2
12	Asks whether the patient takes regular painkillers.	0	1	2

1. The pain of a migraine is unilateral (heMIcrania).
   Tension-type headaches are usually bilateral.
   Pain localised over the temporal area is a feature of temporal arteritis.
   Pain behind the eyes or over the cheeks and forehead occurs in acute sinusitis.
   Pain in the face can be caused by trigeminal neuralgia, temporomandibular arthritis, glaucoma, cluster headache or psychiatric disease.

2. Sinusitis tends to produce a sensation of fullness behind the eyes and over the cheeks, rather than pain.
   Temporal arteritis produces an exquisitely tender area over the temporal artery.
   Tension headaches are often described as a sensation of band-like tightness.

3. A severe headache of sudden onset may be a subarachnoid haemorrhage.
   A subacute onset is suggestive of an inflammatory cause such as meningitis.
   A headache developing and progressing over weeks or months may be due to a mass lesion, especially if other focal neurological features are present.
   Recurring generalised headaches with a history going back several years or months and associated with stress may be tension headaches.
   In headaches of short duration, sinusitis, glaucoma and migrainous neuralgia should be considered.

4. Headache secondary to mass lesions often becomes worse after lying down for a few hours and is present on waking. These headaches are also made worse by coughing or straining.
    In migraine with aura there is usually photophobia.

5. Cluster headaches are typically unilateral and last for hours, occurring in bouts that last several weeks a few times a year. This pattern is more common in males.
    Tension headaches are also episodic, lasting for hours and recurring frequently.

6. Severity is subjective but typically, very severe headaches are suggestive of subarachnoid haemorrhage, meningitis or migraine.
    Tension and cluster headaches are not usually severe enough to wake the patient from sleep.

7. Migraine with aura is classically preceded by the sensation of flashing lights.
    Temporal arteritis may be associated with blurred vision.
    The headache of benign intracranial hypertension can cause visual loss on bending and rising.

8. Vomiting often accompanies the headache of raised intracranial pressure.

9. Haemorrhagic strokes are usually associated with a headache.

10. The headache of meningitis is associated with fever, neck stiffness and photophobia as well as vomiting.
    Subarachnoid haemorrhage leads to meningism (neck stiffness and vomiting).
    Cluster headaches may be associated with lacrimation, rhinorrhoea and flushing of the forehead.

11. Stress is a trigger for tension-type headaches.

12. Analgesia misuse is a very common cause of chronic daily headache.

Presenting Complaint - Sudden Onset Weakness

		Not attempted	Attempted inadequate	Attempted adequate
1	Asks the patient to describe exactly what happened.	0	1	2
2	Asks the patient about the time course of the weakness.	0	1	2
3	Asks the patient whether they fell to the ground.	0	1	2
4	Asks the patient whether they lost consciousness.	0	1	2
5	Asks whether the weakness was confined to one side or affected both and whether facial muscles were affected.	0	1	2
6	Asks about history of headaches and whether the onset of this episode was associated with a headache.	0	1	2
7	Asks whether they noticed any visual disturbance.	0	1	2
8	Asks whether they noticed any speech disturbance.	0	1	2
9	Asks the patient whether they have experienced any similar episodes before.	0	1	2
10	Asks the patient whether they have a history of arrhythmias, MI, hypertension, angina, high cholesterol, diabetes or pain in their calves on exercise.	0	1	2
11	Asks whether the patient takes anticoagulant medication.	0	1	2
12	Asks the patient whether they smoke.	0	1	2

1. A single episode of weakness often represents a TIA or a stroke but it is important to get a clear description of the event as the patient could be describing a seizure or a hypoglycaemic episode.

2. Strokes and TIAs are sudden onset phenomena by definition. However, in TIAs, symptoms reach their peak in seconds and resolve within 24 hours whereas in stroke, symptoms persist.

3. This provides information as to the site of the weakness and also warns about other possible injuries.

4. Loss of consciousness is not a common feature of TIAs or stroke but can occur if the brainstem is affected.

5. This gives clues to the site of the lesion.

6. A haemorrhagic stroke is usually accompanied by a severe headache.
Migraine with a focal prodrome can cause diagnostic confusion with TIAs but TIAs are not usually associated with headaches.
Mass lesions can also cause events similar to TIAs, and may be a cause of headache.

7. Amaurosis fugax is the sudden transient loss of vision in one eye due to involvement of the ipsilateral ophthalmic artery.
   TIAs affecting the posterior circulation can lead to diplopia.
   Brainstem infarction can produce a pattern of diplopia and hemi or tetraparesis with crossed signs.

8. Dysphasia is a common feature of TIAs and of stroke affecting the dominant side of the cortex.

9. TIAs have a tendency to recur and to herald thromboembolic stroke.

10. Atrial fibrillation is a risk factor for thromboembolic infarction.
    Patients who have had an MI are at risk of cerebral embolism.
    Those with a history of coronary or peripheral vascular disease are likely to also have atherosclerosis of their cerebral vessels.
    Hypertension is a risk factor for cerebral haemorrhage.

11. Anticoagulants are a risk factor for haemorrhagic stroke.

12. Smoking is one of the key modifiable risk factors for stroke.

Presenting Complaint - Collapse

		Not attempted	Attempted inadequate	Attempted adequate
1	Asks the patient when the episode(s) occurred.	0	1	2
2	Asks what situation the patient was in at the time.	0	1	2
3	Asks the patient to describe how they felt before they collapsed.	0	1	2
4	Asks whether the patient actually lost consciousness and how long they were unconscious for.	0	1	2
5	Asks whether anyone witnessed the episode and gets them to describe exactly what they saw.	0	1	2
6	Asks whether the patient was incontinent or bit their tongue during the episode.	0	1	2
7	Asks whether the patient banged their head or sustained any other injuries.	0	1	2
8	Asks how the patient felt when they came around from the episode.	0	1	2
9	Asks how the patient feels now, particularly whether they have any problems with speech, vision or with moving their arms or legs.	0	1	2
10	Asks if they have ever experienced a similar episode before.	0	1	2
11	Asks if there is any history of cardiac disease.	0	1	2
12	Asks if the patient ever feels dizzy or weak on standing up from a sitting or lying position.	0	1	2
13	If the patient is a young female, asks if there is any possibility that she could be pregnant and whether she had any abdominal pain or vaginal bleeding.	0	1	2
14	Asks if the patient is diabetic, and if so, asks when they last ate.	0	1	2
15	Asks if the patient has ever had a severe head injury.	0	1	2
16	Asks if the patient takes any medications.	0	1	2
17	Asks if the patient has taken any non-prescription drugs or if they were drinking heavily.	0	1	2
18	Asks whether the patient drives a motor vehicle.	0	1	2

1. It is important to establish how long ago the event occurred so that the patient's current clinical state can be judged in context.

2. Situational or vasovagal syncope may be provoked by fright, anxiety, postural changes, micturition or coughing.
    Exertional syncope may occur if there is obstruction to the left ventricular outflow by aortic stenosis or cardiac myopathy.
    Flickering lights and alcohol can be triggers for seizures.

3. A vasovagal syncope is often preceded by a prodrome of nausea, dizziness, tinnitus, blurred / grey vision and sweating.
    If the collapse followed an arrhythmia, the patient may have felt palpitations or chest pain before the event but it may have occurred without warning.
    Patients with hypoglycaemia may report sweating, weakness and confusion before losing consciousness.
    Seizures may be preceded by an aura, the form of which depends on the area of brain affected, or may have no prodrome.

4. Syncope involves loss of consciousness by definition. Vasovagal syncope often lasts no more than a few seconds. Cardiovascular syncope is also usually brief but the patient is typically deeply unconscious and very pale for its duration.
    Falls without loss of consciousness are common in Parkinson's disease and are the hallmark of drop attacks.
    If the patient has had a seizure, loss or impairment of consciousness helps to classify seizure type. If consciousness is impaired, the seizure is described as complex whereas if it is unimpaired, the seizure is described as simple.

5. A witness history is important in these cases.
    A few jerky movements may occur in a vasovagal episode, particularly if the patient is prevented from getting into a supine position (eg. held up by bystanders). This is termed anoxic syncopal seizure.
    A generalised seizure is often preceded by a cry and then consists of tonic-clonic movements often with cyanosis and frothing at the mouth.
    Cardiac syncopal events are abrupt in onset and often accompanied by pallor and sweating.

6. Incontinence can occur in syncope and in seizures. Tongue-biting is very suggestive of a tonic-clonic seizure.

7. It is important to know whether the patient has any physical injuries.

8. Recovery from a cardiac syncope is usually rapid with flushing and deep / sighing respiration in some cases.
    Recovery from a vaso-vagal episode is usually rapid and complete.
    Post-ictal drowsiness or confusion is normal following a generalised seizure - rapid recovery should lead you to question the diagnosis.

9. TIAs or strokes can cause collapse associated with cognitive, motor or sensory symptoms.

10. Epilepsy is the continuing tendency to have seizures. In those patients with diagnosed epilepsy, try to establish why the seizure might have occurred this time. Common reasons for decreased control include poor compliance with medication, intercurrent illness, alcohol or drug ingestion.
    Elderly patients in particular may have a history of falls that need investigating.

11. Patients with collapse due to arrhythmias may have a history of MI, cardiomyopathy or valvular disease.
Severe aortic stenosis is associated with exertional syncope.

12. These are symptoms of postural hypotension which needs to be investigated (it could be due to autonomic neuropathy or hypovolaemia).

13. Collapse associated with abdominal pain should alert you to the possibility of an ectopic pregnancy.

14. Hypoglycaemic episodes can occur in diabetics on insulin therapy if they miss a meal or snack or over-exert themselves unexpectedly.

15. A head injury can be followed by epilepsy in the first week or many months or years later. To cause epilepsy the injury usually has to have been significant enough to cause loss of consciousness.

16. Nitrates, antihypertensives, tricyclics and antiarrhythmics are all commonly implicated in falls / collapse.

17. Drugs and alcohol are common causes of collapse.

18. It is illegal to drive a motor vehicle if any unexplained loss of consciousness has occurred in the previous year and it is an essential requirement of doctors to inform patients of these regulations.

Examination Of The Cranial Nerves

		Not attempted	Attempted inadequate	Attempted adequate
1	Approaches the patient politely and introduces himself/herself.	0	1	2
2	Performs a general inspection of the head and neck commenting on scars, neurofibromas, facial asymmetry, ptosis, proptosis, skew deviation of the eyes or inequality of the pupils.	0	1	2
3	Tests the sense of smell in each nostril separately using a series of smell test bottles.	0	1	2
4	Tests the visual acuity of each eye separately using a Snellen chart.	0	1	2
5	Tests for visual inattention by asking the patient to report whether the examiner's finger is moving on one side or both sides simultaneously.	0	1	2
6	Tests for visual field defects in each eye separately by confrontation.	0	1	2
7	Tests direct and consensual pupil responses to light, asking the patient to look straight ahead and bringing the pen torch in from the side. Performs the swinging light test.	0	1	2
8	Asks the patient to focus on a distant point and then on the examiner's finger held 30cm in front of their nose. Comments on any abnormality in accomodation.	0	1	2
9	Examines the fundi using an ophthalmoscope.	0	1	2
10	Tests eye movements in all directions, asking the patient to report any double vision. Comments on any failure of movement or nystagmus.	0	1	2
11	Tests superficial sensation in the three divisions of the trigeminal nerve by asking the patient to close their eyes and indicating when they feel the cotton wool touching them. Compares the divisions on either side of the face.	0	1	2
12	Test deep sensation in the three divisions of the trigeminal nerve by asking the patient to close their eyes and indicating whether they feel a pin prick as sharp or dull (the examiner should first demonstrate the two sensations by touching the skin over the sternum). Compares the divisions on either side of the face.	0	1	2
13	Tests the corneal reflex.	0	1	2
14	Asks the patient to clench their teeth and	0	1	2

	feels the masseter muscles. Asks the patient to open their mouth and not to let it be closed by the examiner's force.			
15	Tests the jaw-jerk reflex.	0	1	2
16	Tests the muscles of facial expression (asks the patient to screw up their eyes and not to let them be opened, blow out their cheeks, raise their eyebrows, purse their lips, grin and show the examiner their teeth). Asks if the patient has experienced any changes in their hearing.	0	1	2
17	Tests the hearing by whispering a number into each ear at a time and asking the patient to repeat it. Asks the patient if they have experienced any dizziness or had trouble with their balance.	0	1	2
18	Looks at the palate commenting on any uveal displacement. Ask the patient to say 'ah' and comments on any asymmetry of movement. Asks whether the patient has any difficulty swallowing. Performs the gag reflex.	0	1	2
19	Asks the patient to shrug their shoulders and attempts to push them down. Asks the patient to turn their head against resistance and feels sternomastoid. Repeats for the other sternomastoid.	0	1	2
20	Looks at the tongue when it is relaxed in the mouth, commenting on any fasciculation or wasting.	0	1	2
21	Asks the patient to stick out their tongue and comments on any deviation. Asks the patient to push their tongue into their cheek against resistance of the examiner's finger.	0	1	2
22	Thanks patient and washes hands			

1. It is important to introduce yourself (give your name and what you do) and explain that you are to examine their nervous system. Explain what you are going to do as you proceed with the examination, *before* you do it!

2. A general inspection can reveal a pattern of abnormalities, which may be missed when each cranial nerve is examined separately.

3. Olfactory nerve (CN I).
   This is usually only tested if the patient complains of loss of sense of smell. If the patient is able to identify a scent, that is all that's needed. If they can't identify it, ask them whether it is different from the next scent offered.
   A loss of the sense of smell is most commonly caused by upper respiratory tract infection but in the absence of this may be due to a meningioma in the olfactory groove or a basal or frontal skull fracture.

4. Optic nerve (CN II)
   If the patient usually wears glasses or contact lenses visual acuity should be assessed with these in place.
   The patient should be positioned 6m from a Snellen chart. Count the number of whole lines that they can read.
   Decreased visual acuity can be due to conditions affecting the eye itself (such as glaucoma, macular degeneration, diabetic retinopathy or cataracts) or due to lesions affecting the optic nerve, chiasma, tract or cortex (such as trauma, infarction or tumours).

5. Optic nerve (CN II)
   Ask the patient to look directly at you.
   Hold your fingers up in the periphery of their visual field and waggle your fingertip on one side at a time and then both sides together, asking the patient to report which side is moving.
   If there is inattention, the patient will be able to detect movement on both sides individually but will ignore one side when there is movement in both simultaneously.
   Test this in both upper and lower quadrants.

6. Optic nerve (CN II)
   It is important that your eye level is the same as the patient's and that they look straight into your eyes. The eye not being tested should be covered.
   Bring a white pin into the visual field from the periphery and by asking them to say when they see it, compare their visual fields to yours. Test each quadrant in turn in both eyes.
   Total unilateral visual loss is due to a lesion of the optic nerve or to unilateral eye disease.
   A bitemporal hemianopia is caused by a lesion affecting the centre of the optic chiasm, commonly a pituitary tumour.
   A homonymous hemianopia is caused by a lesion affecting anywhere between the optic tract and the occipital cortex eg. a tumour or a haemorrhage.

7. Optic nerve (CN II)
   The light source should always be brought in from the side so that the patient does not focus on it and accommodate.
   The swinging light test is performed by moving a torch in an arc from pupil to pupil. It is used to test for an abnormality in the afferent pathway, eg. due to optic atrophy. When the light is shone on the normal side, the contralateral pupil constricts; the consensual response. However, when the light is swung to the abnormal side, the pupil paradoxically dilates, as the direct response on that side is weaker than the consensual one.

8. Optic nerve (CN II)
   A normal accommodation response involves constriction of both pupils.
   Neurosyphilis characteristically leads to a pupil, which will accommodate but doesn't react to light (an Argyll Robertson pupil).

9. This should be done as part of the routine examination of the cranial nerves.

10. Oculomotor (CN III), trochlear (CN IV) and abducens (CN VI) nerves.
    Ask the patient to hold their head steady and follow the movement of your finger.
    Make an H shape and then an I shape in the centre.
    Abnormal eye movement may be due to a central lesion, a muscular condition, a III, IV or VI nerve palsy (see below for specifics) or to an abnormality of the orbit.
    Diplopia is a sign of ocular muscle weakness. The false image is the peripheral one.

Nystagmus is normal at the extremes of gaze. Nystagmus present with the eyes in any other position can be caused by many conditions including multiple sclerosis, vestibular or cerebellar lesions and toxins.
If any abnormality is detected further testing is needed.

Lesions of CN III are usually idiopathic or following trauma, although the nerve can be affected by tumours, ischaemia or demyelination. CN III supplies the superior, medial and inferior rectii, inferior oblique and levator palpebrae superioris and it is accompanied by parasympathetic fibres to the pupil. Lesions therefore result in ptosis, an eye pointing down and out and a fixed and dilated pupil.

Isolated lesions to CN IV are rare (they are usually associated with CN III palsies). They result in diplopia when the patient tries to look downwards and away from the affected side as CN IV supplies superior oblique.

Lesions to CN VI most often occur following trauma or Wernicke's encephalopathy. They lead to failure of lateral movement, convergent strabismus and diplopia as CN VI supplies lateral rectus.

11. Trigeminal nerve (CN V).
    If an area of reduced sensation is detected, the boundaries should be mapped. Total sensory loss in all 3 divisions suggests that the lesion is at the level of the ganglion or at the sensory root. Loss of sensation in one division, suggests a post-ganglionic lesion.

12. Again, map out the area of any altered sensation.

13. Trigeminal (CN V) and facial (CN VII) nerves.
    The cornea should be lightly touched with cotton wool brought in from the side. If the reflex is intact, both eyes will blink. The sensory component of the reflex is carried by the ophthalmic division of the trigeminal nerve but the motor component is carried by the facial nerve. Failure of the reflex means that an abnormality in either of these nerves is a possibility.

14. Trigeminal nerve (CN V).
    The muscles of mastication are supplied by the motor component of the trigeminal nerve. A unilateral lesion will cause the jaw to deviate towards the side of the lesion.

15. Trigeminal nerve (CN V).
    The patient should let their mouth fall open slightly and the examiner's finger should be placed on their jaw and tapped lightly with a tendon hammer. The normal response is slight or absent. An exaggerated response implies an upper motor neurone lesion and is often seen in pseudobulbar palsy.

16. Facial nerve (CN VII).
    This is the motor supply to the muscles of facial expression.
    A LMN lesion leads to weakness of all the muscles of facial expression on the same side as the lesion. There are a number of causes but the most common form is a Bell's palsy which is idiopathic.
    An UMN lesion also results in ipsilateral weakness of the muscles of facial expression but spares the forehead. This is because the frontalis muscle has a bilateral cortical supply. UMN lesions are most commonly caused by tumours or vascular events.
    CN VII also carries the motor supply to stapedius. Damage to the nerve paralyses the muscle leading to hyperacusis (unpleasantly loud distortion of sounds).

17. Vestibulocochlear nerve (CN VIII).
   The opposite ear should be covered whilst a number is whispered.
   This is a crude test and if any abnormality is suspected, the patient should be referred for formal hearing testing.
   Deafness can be classified into conduction deafness or sensorineural deafness. Causes of conduction deafness include wax, otitis media, otosclerosis and Paget's disease of bone. Causes of sensorineural deafness include environmental exposure to noise, tumours, infection, Meniere's disease and effects of drugs eg. aspirin and gentamicin.
   Vertigo can be caused by Meniere's disease, vestibular neuronitis and brainstem lesions.

18. Glossopharyngeal (IX) and vagus (X) nerves.
   The glossopharyngeal nerve carries sensory fibres from the pharynx and posterior third of the tongue. The vagus nerve carries the sensory supply from the pharynx and larynx and innervates muscles of the pharynx, larynx and palate. Combined lesions of CN IX and X therefore lead to difficulty swallowing, nasal regurgitation and choking.
   The uvula is drawn to the normal side in a CN X palsy.
   To detect the gag reflex, depress the tongue and touch the back of the throat with an orange stick. Use a pen torch to observe the response. The sensory component of the reflex is carried by CN IX and the motor component by CN X. A normal response is contraction of the soft palate. The reflex decreases with age.

19. Accessory nerve (XI).
   The spinal division carries the motor supply to trapezius and sternomastoid.
   The right sternomastoid turns the head to the left.
   A unilateral CN XI lesion can be caused by trauma to the neck or base of the skull.
   A bilateral CN XI lesion can be caused by motor neurone disease, or the Guillan-Barre syndrome.

20. Hypoglossal nerve (XII).
   Wasting or fasciculations indicate a LMN lesion.

21. Hypoglossal nerve (XII).
   If there is a unilateral LMN lesion, the tongue will deviate towards the affected side.
   This has many possible causes both central and peripheral.
   An UMN lesion of CN XII is usually only noticeable when it is bilateral in which case, it results in a small, immobile tongue. It is most commonly caused by tumour, motor neurone disease or vascular lesions.

22. It is polite to thank the patient. Always wash and disinfect your hands to reduce the risk of cross-infection.

Neurological Examination Of The Lower Limbs

		Not attempted	Attempted inadequate	Attempted adequate
1	Approaches the patient politely and introduces himself/herself. Exposes the patient adequately after obtaining their permission	0	1	2
2	Inspects the lower limbs for muscle wasting, fasciculation or deformity.	0	1	2
3	Tests tone at the knee and ankle in both limbs by passively bending the joints in an unexpected and irregular fashion. Tests for clonus at the ankle.	0	1	2
4	Tests power at both hip joints.	0	1	2
5	Tests power at both knee joints.	0	1	2
6	Tests power at both ankle joints.	0	1	2
7	Tests the knee jerk reflex.	0	1	2
8	Tests the ankle reflex.	0	1	2
9	Tests the plantar reflex.	0	1	2
10	Tests co-ordination with a suitable test (e.g. heel-knee test).	0	1	2
11	Tests superficial sensation in each dermatome on both limbs.	0	1	2
12	Tests deep sensation in each dermatome on both limbs.	0	1	2
13	Tests proprioception at a DIP joint in each foot, and successive joints working up the limb if any deficit is detected.	0	1	2
14	Tests vibration sense at a DIP joint in each foot, and successive joints up the limb if any deficit is detected, using a 128Hz tuning fork.	0	1	2
15	Performs Romberg's test.	0	1	2
16	Assesses gait by asking the patient to walk normally first, then heel-to-toe, then on their toes and then on their heels.	0	1	2
17	Thanks patient and washes hands			

1. It is important to introduce yourself (give your name and what you do) and explain that you are to examine their nerve supply to the legs. Explain that you need to expose their legs fully in order to perform an adequate examination. Respect the modesty of patients. Explain what you are going to do as you proceed with the examination, *before* you do it!

2. Muscle wasting indicates disuse atrophy, primary muscle disease or denervation. Always consider the pattern of wasting ie. proximal or distal, symmetrical or asymmetrical.
Fasciculations are usually benign if there are no other signs of motor abnormality. If associated with weakness or wasting, fasciculations suggest a LMN problem eg. peripheral neuropathy. They can also occur in primary myopathy and thryotoxicosis. Deformity implies a chronic condition. Pes cavus is a sign of long standing problems with foot innervation.

3. The patient needs to be relaxed for this.
    Test for tone in the knee by placing one hand under the knee and suddenly flicking it up causing flexion. If the ankle lifts of the bed, this implies increased tone.
    At the ankle, tone can be assessed by supporting the lower leg and passively flexing and extending the joint in an irregular fashion.
    UMN lesions lead to hypertonia whereas LMN lesions lead to hypotonia.
    Clonus at the ankle is elicited by sharply dorsiflexing the foot whilst supporting the limb with the knee flexed and the thigh externally rotated. A few beats of plantar flexion of the ankle can be normal but sustained clonus is characteristic of an UMN lesion.

4. Power at each joint should be rated on the Medical Research Council scale of   0-5:
    5 = normal power
    4 = reduced power against resistance
    3 = movement against gravity but not resistance
    2 = movement when gravity is eliminated e.g. if the leg is supported on the bed, they can adduct it.
    1 = flicker of contraction
    0 = paralysis

    Painful joint and muscle conditions can interfere with the assessment of power.

    Iliop-psoas (L1, 2), hip flexion:
    Ask them to lift their leg up, holding it straight, and to stop you pushing it down.
    Gluteus maximus (L5, S1, 2), hip extension:
    Ask them to keep their leg down whilst you try and elevate it from under their calf.

5. Hamstrings (L5, S1, 2), knee flexion:
    Ask them to bend their knee and not to let you straighten it.
    Quadriceps (L2, 3, 4), knee extension:
    Ask them to try and resist you bending their knee further.

6. Tibialis anterior (L4,5), ankle dorsiflexion:
    Ask them to resist you plantar flexing their ankle.
    Gastrocnemius and soleus (S1, 2), ankle plantar flexion:
    Ask them to resist you dorsiflexing their ankle.

7. Knee jerk (L3, 4):
    Support the knee so that it is slightly bent and tap over the infrapatellar tendon with the tendon hammer.
    If any reflex appears to be absent, ask the patient to clench their teeth or to interlock their fingers and pull apart hard as you are testing for the reflex.

8. Ankle jerk (S1, 2):
    Externally rotate the leg, flex the knee and dorsiflex the foot. Tap the tendon.
    On their left side, it is easier to use a backhanded motion.
    An alternative approach to assessing this reflex is to get the patient to kneel with their feet hanging over the edge of the bed.

9. Plantar reflex (L5, S1, 2):
    Stroke the lateral aspect of the sole of the foot with a blunt object.
    The normal response is flexion of the big toe at the MTP joint with flexion and adduction of the other toes.
    An upgoing (Babinski) response indicates that there is an UMN lesion.

10. Ask the patient to close their eyes and place their heel on their opposite knee, running it down their leg to their foot. A patient with cerebellar disease will struggle to do this, with the heel oscillating from side to side and overshooting.
Coordination will also be abnormal in UMN lesions due to weakness and spasticity.

11. Touch an area of skin from each dermatome with a wisp of cotton wool, asking the patient to keep their eyes closed and indicate when they feel the touch. Compare dermatomes on either limb.
Don't stroke the skin as this moves hairs.
If any area of abnormal sensation is detected, map out the boundaries by going from the abnormal towards the normal area.

> Upper thigh = L2
> Anterior knee = L3
> Inner calf = L4
> Outer calf = L5
> Lateral foot = S1

12. Demonstrate the sharp and blunt feel of either end of the pin to the patient by touching it over their sternum.
Test each dermatome in turn, asking the patient to say whether they feel the pin as sharp or blunt. Compare sides and map out any area of abnormality.

13. Hold the great toe by the lateral aspects and demonstrate up and down movements to the patient. Then ask them to **close their eyes** and say whether the movement is up or down as you move the joint randomly. Make the movements as small as possible initially.

14. Ask the patient to close their eyes. Place a vibrating tuning fork (128Hz) on one of their DIP joints and ask them to indicate when they feel you deaden the vibrations.

15. Ask the patient to stand with their feet together. Once they are stable, ask them to close their eyes. If unsteadiness increases, Romberg's test is positive. It is associated with a loss of proprioception.

16. Heel-to-toe walking tests for a midline cerebellar lesion.
An S1 lesion leads to difficulty in walking on their toes.
An L4 / L5 lesion leads to difficulty in walking on their heels (footdrop).

Common neurological patterns of gait disturbance include:
- Spasticity - stiff and jerky on a narrow base.
- Parkinson's disease - hesitation in starting, shuffling, freezing, festination, propulsion, retropulsion and diminished swinging of the arms.
- Cerebellar ataxia - broad-based, unstable and tremulous. The gait veers towards the side of the more affected cerebellar lobe.
- Sensory ataxia - broad-based and high stepping.
- Distal weakness - the affected leg has to be lifted high and the foot returns to the ground with an audible slap.
- Proximal weakness - waddling.
- Hemiplegia - plantar flexed foot with leg swung in lateral arc.

Joint and muscle problems can also alter the gait.

17. . It is polite to thank the patient. Always wash and disinfect your hands to reduce the risk of cross-infection.

Neurological Examination Of The Upper Limbs

		Not attempted	Attempted inadequate	Attempted adequate
1	Approaches the patient politely and introduces himself/herself. Exposes the patient adequately after obtaining their permission	0	1	2
2	Inspects the upper limbs for muscle wasting, tremor, fasciculation and deformities.	0	1	2
3	Asks the patient to hold out both hands, palms facing upwards, with the arms extended and the eyes closed. Comments on any drift.	0	1	2
4	Tests tone at the elbow and wrist in both arms by passively bending the joints in an unexpected and irregular fashion. Comments on supinator catch and cogwheel rigidity.	0	1	2
5	Tests power at both shoulder joints.	0	1	2
6	Tests power at the elbow joints in both arms.	0	1	2
7	Tests power at the wrist joint in both arms	0	1	2
8	Tests power at the finger joints in both hands.	0	1	2
9	Tests the biceps reflex.	0	1	2
10	Tests the triceps reflex.	0	1	2
11	Tests the supinator reflex.	0	1	2
12	Tests co-ordination with a suitable test (eg. finger-nose test, testing for dysdiadochokinesis etc.).	0	1	2
13	Tests superficial sensation in each dermatome on both limbs.	0	1	2
14	Tests deep sensation in each dermatome on both limbs.	0	1	2
15	Tests proprioception at a DIP joint in each hand, and successive joints working up the limb if any deficit is detected.	0	1	2
16	Tests vibration sense at a DIP joint in each limb, and successive joints up the limb if any deficit is detected, using a 128Hz tuning fork.	0	1	2
17	Thanks patient and washes hands			

1. It is important to introduce yourself (give your name and what you do) and explain that you would like to examine their arms. Explain what you are going to do as you proceed with the examination, *before* you do it!

2. See point 2 of examination of the lower limbs.

3. There are 3 causes of arm drift:

An UMN lesion - the drift is due to weakness and tends to be in the downward and medial direction. The forearm pronates and the fingers may flex.
Cerebellar disease - the drift is due to hypotonia and is upwards.
Loss of proprioception - the drift can be in any direction.

4. Support the patient's elbow with one hand and hold their hand with the other.
Assess tone during flexion, extension, pronation and supination.
A supinator catch is characteristic of increased tone and is easily detected by rapid rotation of the forearm.
Cogwheel rigidity occurs in Parkinson's disease. There is increased tone which gives way in a series of jerks. If hypertonia is not easy to detect, ask the patient to open and close the fist of the other hand to reinforce any increased tone in the wrist that you are moving.

5. Deltoid (C5, 6):
Ask the patient to hold their arms abducted and flexed at the elbow (chicken wings) and not to let you push them down.
Latissimus dorsi and pectoralis major (C6, 7, 8), shoulder adduction:
With their arms in the same position, ask the patient to resist you lifting their arms up further.

6. Biceps (C5, 6), elbow flexion:
Ask the patient to bend their elbows to about 90° and not to let you straighten them.
Triceps (C7), elbow extension:
Ask them to resist you bending their arms further.

7. Flexor carpi radialis and ulnaris (C6, 7, 8,), wrist flexion:
Support under the patient's forearm. Ask them not to let you extend their wrists.
Extensor carpi radialis (C7, 8), wrist extension:
Support under the patient's forearm. Ask them not to let you flex their wrists.

8. Flexor digitorum profundus and superficialis (C7, 8), finger flexion:
Ask them to squeeze your fingers.
Extensor digitorum (C7, 8), finger extension:
Support under the palm. Ask them to keep their fingers straight and not to let you push them down.
Dorsal interossei (C8, T1):
Ask them to spread their fingers apart and not to let you push them together. The Dorsal interossei ABduct (DAB).
Palmer interossei (C8, T1):
Ask them to hold their fingers tightly together and not to let you pull them apart. The Palmar interossei ADduct (PAD).

9. Biceps reflex (C5, 6):
Ask the patient to sit comfortably with the elbows flexed and the hands lying pronated in their lap. Place a finger over the biceps tendon first and tap that rather than tapping the tendon directly.

10. Triceps reflex (C7, 8):
For this, the patient's arm needs to be positioned further across their body. Tap the tendon directly.

11. Supinator reflex (C5, 6):
With the patient's arms relaxed in their lap, place your thumb over the brachioradialis tendon on the radial side of the forearm, just above the wrist. Tap your thumb and observe for flexion of the elbow.

12. Perform the finger-nose test by holding your finger just less than an arm's length away from them and asking them to touch your finger, then their nose. Move the target during the patient's attempts. Repeat the process with them using the other hand.

    Intention tremor and past pointing are indicative of cerebellar disease.

    Another test of coordination is to ask them to hold one hand flat, palm up and turn the other hand over repeatedly on it as fast as they can. An inability to do this is known as dysdiadochokinesis and is another characteristic feature of cerebellar disease.

13. See point 11 of examination of the lower limbs for how to test for sensation.

    Outer aspect of upper arm = C5
    Lateral aspect of forearm and thumb = C6
    Middle finger = C7
    Little finger = C8
    Medial aspect of upper arm = T1

14. See point 12 of examination of the lower limbs.

15. See point 13 of examination of the lower limbs.

16. See point 14 of examination of the lower limbs.
17. It is polite to thank the patient. Always wash your hands to reduce the risk of cross-infection.

Cognitive State Assessment

		Not attempted	Attempted inadequate	Attempted adequate
1	Approaches the patient politely and introduces him/herself.	0	1	2
2	Checks the patient's name and explains what the interview is about.	0	1	2
3	Asks the patient if they have been having any problems recently, particularly with their memory.	0	1	2
4	Tests immediate recall.	0	1	2
5	Tests orientation for time, person and place.	0	1	2
6	Tests concentration and attention e.g using serial 7s.	0	1	2
7	Tests recent long term memory.	0	1	2
8	Tests remote long term memory.	0	1	2
9	Tests short term memory.	0	1	2
10	Thanks the patient and invites any questions from them.	0	1	2

1. It is polite to introduce yourself.
2. It is especially important in this situation to explain why you are seeing the patient and what you are going to do. Try to put the patient at ease.
3. Ask a one or two general, open questions initially to gauge the patient's understanding and assessment of the problem.
4. Give the patient a name and address to remember and ask them to repeat it back immediately. Explain that you are also going to ask them for it again at the end. If they cannot repeat it immediately, repeat the whole thing and ask them to try it again. Use a maximum of three attempts. If they are unable to manage the address, ask them to recall three unrelated objects.
5. Time - ask what year it is currently. Person - ask if they know who you are. Place - ask the patient where they are at the moment. Ask for detail such as building, town, county and country.
6. Ask them to start at 100 and take away 7 repeatedly until you ask them to stop. If they are unable to do serial 7s, then ask for the days of the week in reverse order.
7. Tailor this to the age of the patient and their culture / hobbies. For example, ask if they keep up with the news and then ask them about something that has been happening recently.
8. Again, tailor this to age and culture. For example, ask whether they know the dates of the beginning and end of world war II.
9. Ask if they can remember the address that you gave them about three minutes ago.
10. Be prepared to give an assessment of your findings in a tactful and reassuring manner.

Top Tips

Neurological Examination

Under exam conditions, being polite and courteous to patients will always score highly, so make sure that they are comfortable and always cover them once the exam is over.

Exam technique - the keys are familiarity and repetition

Neurological cases are common in finals, because the signs are striking and static. You will not be asked to examine the entire nervous system. Instead, be prepared to assess cranial nerves, limbs, gait, speech, or higher mental functions. Looking hard before acting may reveal a huge amount (obvious facial palsy? Fasciculations? Walking stick?).

The abbreviated mental test.

Ask your patient:

- How old are you?

- What time is it? (to the nearest hour)

- Where do you live?

- Where are you? (They should respond with the name of the hospital)

- To identify two people

- What is your date of birth?

- In which year was the end of the second world war?

- Who is the monarch?

- To count backwards from 20 to 1

Another version:

Orientation: What is the year, season, date, day and/or month?

Where are we? Country, County, City, Hospital

Registration: Name three objects slowly. Then ask patient to repeat them all together back to you.

Recall: Ask patient to remember a sequence and repeat it after an interval.

Language: Read and obey a command

Follow a 3-stage command (e.g., pick up pencil/put down paper/fold paper)

Ask patient to copy a complex diagram

Cranial nerves

A cranial nerve examination can be done in under a minute, by practising the routine hundreds of times on family and friends. Any deviation from this routine is usually startling. Always compare left with right.

When you see a sign, it is sometimes hard to remember where the pathology lies. A unilateral palsy of the glossopharyngeal or vagus nerves (IX and X) causes the palate to move away from the affected side when the patient says "Aah." In contrast, a unilateral lesion of the hypoglossal nerve causes the tongue to deviate towards the affected side when it is protruded. So: "Palate away, tongue towards".

Limbs

Examining the limbs is not synonymous with examining the peripheral nervous system, since you will be assessing aspects of both upper and lower motor neurone function. Again, be comparative, so assess tone in one arm, then in the other, before moving on to power.

Gait

Ask the patient to stand with his/her eyes open, then closed, to walk, turn around, walk on his/her heels and then his/her toes. In a spastic gait the patient drags his/her affected leg, with the foot plantar flexed and inverted, and the toes scuffing the ground (fig 2). The Parkinsonian gait is shuffling, with difficulty initiating movements and turning. An ataxic gait is unsteady and broad based, and it can be exaggerated by asking the patient to walk heel-toe as if on a tightrope. The two main causes of gait ataxia are cerebellar disease and sensory loss. In the latter, the patient relies on being able to see and place his feet as s/he walks, since s/he is missing positional feedback. If s/he closes his/her eyes, his/her unsteadiness worsens - this is a positive Romberg's sign. In a foot drop, owing to a lateral popliteal nerve palsy or L5 root lesion, the patient has to lift the affected foot high off the ground, and it returns with a distinctive "slap."

Speech

Your routine questions should distinguish between dysphonia (poor voice production), dysarthria (a mechanical disorder of articulation) and dysphasia (a language or communication disorder). Remember that we are all temporarily dysarthric, but not dysphasic, after a visit to the dentist or the pub. Examiners are impressed if you can distinguish between a receptive dysphasia, where comprehension is impaired, and an expressive type where it remains intact, although they usually coexist.

Begin a conversation with your patient, perhaps by asking his/her name and address, and listen for clues. If his/her speech sounds dysarthric, this sign can be exaggerated by asking him/her to say something complicated ("West Register Street"). Next, ask him/her to obey a simple command - which will be difficult if s/he has a receptive dysphasia. A common expressive dysphasia entails difficulty in naming objects (nominal dysphasia), so point to your pen or tie and ask what it is. You can confirm an isolated expressive problem by giving a range of possibilities: "Is it a torch? Is it a hammer? Is it a pen?" and the patient will nod appropriately.

Higher mental functions

In your medical finals, a simple 10 point mental test will suffice. Learn one by heart, and avoid the Queen's name and the world wars, since they are too culturally specific. You may be asked the causes of acute confusion versus chronic cognitive decline (dementia). In psychiatry exams, be prepared to perform a thorough cognitive assessment - you could use the well known 30 point mini mental state examination.

Localisation - keep it simple

The lesion will be in one (or more) of these places: brain, brain stem, spinal cord, nerve roots, peripheral nerves, neuromuscular junction, muscles.

The most important distinction is between upper and lower motor neurone lesions (table). "Upper" refers to the brain, brain stem, and cord, and the rest is "lower". Keep in mind a patient with a stroke as a paradigm of upper motor neurone signs, with weak and

138

stiff limbs down one side, brisk reflexes, and an extensor plantar. This weakness is said to have a pyramidal tract distribution. In the affected arm the flexors are stronger than the extensors, so the stroke patient holds his arm tightly flexed. In the affected leg the converse is true, with stronger extensors causing the leg to be held out straight. Remember that multiple sclerosis is a disease of the brain and cord, so it only produces upper motor neurone signs.

Comparison of upper and lower neurone lesions

	Upper	Lower
Fasciculations	No	Yes
Wasting	Only if lack of use is prolonged	Yes
Tone	Increased, spastic	Decreased, flaccid
Weakness	Yes	Yes
Reflexes	Exaggerated	Depressed or absent
Clonus	Yes	No
Plantar response	Extensor	Flexor

As a paradigm of lower motor neurone loss, think of a patient with polio - leading to a wasted, fasciculating, flaccid, weak limb. You can further localise peripheral nerve problems by considering if the signs fit a glove and stocking distribution (a peripheral neuropathy - for example, in diabetes mellitus), a single nerve lesion (a mononeuritis - for example, ulnar nerve palsy) or multiple discrete nerve lesions (mononeuritis multiplex - for example, in a vasculitis).

Mixed upper and lower motor neurone lesions are often the result of problems of the cervical cord (with lower motor neurone signs at the level of the lesion, and upper motor neurone signs below it), or motor neurone disease.

If you suspect a spinal cord lesion, you should try and elicit sensory or motor signs that roughly indicate the level.

You should have a basic idea of the functions of different regions of the brain and the clinical consequences of lesions in each, such as personality change and disinhibition in a frontal lobe syndrome . Cerebellar signs are common in exams, and easy to remember (box).

Cerebellar signs - remember the mnemonic DANISH!

- Dysdiadochokinesis

- Ataxia

- Nystagmus

- Intention tremor

- Slurred speech

- Hypotonia

Cerebellar Function Tests:

Heel to Shin

Finger to Nose

Finger to Finger (patient vs doctor)

Rapid Alternating Movements

Learn only a few causes - concentrate on common diseases

If asked for the cause of a cranial nerve lesion, don't mention Wegener's granulomatosis first of all. In fact, all cranial nerve lesions can be caused by trauma, tumours, diabetes mellitus, or multiple sclerosis. Most lists of causes can be stripped down in this way.

In your exam, and in clinical practice, you can predict the commonest conditions. Make sure you have examined patients with stroke, multiple sclerosis, Parkinson's disease, dementia, peripheral and cranial nerve lesions.

Adapted from sBMJ 1999;07 December with permission from the BMJ Publishing Group.

PARKINSONS

Pill rolling tremor
Akinesia
Risidity
Kyphosis
Instability
Neck stiffness
Shuffling gait
Oculogyric crises
Nose tap (glabellar tap)
Small writing

The Musculoskeletal System

Presenting Complaint - Joint Pain

		Not attempted	Attempted inadequate	Attempted adequate
1	Approaches the patient politely and introduces him/herself.	0	1	2
2	Asks the patient's name, DOB and occupation.	0	1	2
3	Asks whether the patient has pain in their joints, muscles or back.	0	1	2
4	Asks whether the pain is associated with swelling or stiffness.	0	1	2
5	Asks how long the symptoms have been going on.	0	1	2
6	Asks if the symptoms are getting worse or staying the same.	0	1	2
7	Asks whether one or many joints are involved.	0	1	2
8	Asks the patient what the sequence of onset of joint involvement was.	0	1	2
9	Asks whether the symptoms are worse at any time of day.	0	1	2
10	If their joints are stiff in the morning, asks how long it takes for the stiffness to wear off.	0	1	2
11	Asks whether the pain ever keeps them awake at night.	0	1	2
12	Asks to what extent the symptoms interfere with the patient's everyday life.	0	1	2
13	Asks whether the patient has injured their joints in the past.	0	1	2
14	Asks whether they have noticed any skin or nail changes.	0	1	2
15	Asks whether the patient has any bowel, eye or urinary symptoms.	0	1	2
16	Asks about relevant past or current conditions including recent infections, psoriasis, inflammatory bowel disease, diabetes, hypertension, osteoporosis and malignancies.	0	1	2
17	Asks about family history of rheumatoid arthritis, gout, osteoarthritis, spondarthritides, psoriasis and inflammatory bowel disease.	0	1	2
18	Asks what medications the patient is on and if they have any allergies to medications.	0	1	2
19	Asks about smoking and alcohol consumption.	0	1	2
20	Asks about home and work circumstances.	0	1	2

1. It is polite to introduce yourself and explain your task.

1. Name: to establish rapport and identify the patient.
   Age/DOB: certain diseases affect certain age groups, e.g. osteoarthritis rarely affects the under 50s whereas rheumatoid arthritis is most common in women aged 30-50 yrs. Back pain under the age of 20 or occurring for the first time over the age of 55 should always be investigated. The date of birth should be recorded to identify the patient.
   Occupation: this can tell you a lot about a person's background and can have significant effects on the management of their condition.

2. Pain in the joints, muscles or back is a common symptom with a large number of underlying causes. It is important to establish exactly where the pain is arising from and to where it radiates.

3. Swelling and stiffness imply that there is inflammation in a joint.

4. Acute symptoms are characteristic of infection or trauma but could be the onset of a chronic problem.
   Chronic symptoms may indicate chronic infection eg. TB, or an underlying condition such as rheumatoid arthritis, one of the spondarthritides (ankylosing spondylitis, psoriatic arthritis, reactive arthritis or enteropathic arthritis) or a connective tissue disease.
   Gout usually presents as an acute episode, which resolves but has a tendency to recur in the same individual.

5. Many rheumatological conditions run a chronic course punctuated by acute exacerbations.

6. The differential diagnosis is different for monoarthritis and polyarthritis.
   Acute monoarthritis is most commonly due to trauma, septic arthritis, gout or pseudogout.
   Chronic monoarthritis is most commonly due to chronic infection or one of the spondarthritides.
   Acute polyarthritis is less common. It can occur in SLE or as part of a para-infectious non-septic arthritis (e.g. hepatitis).
   Chronic polyarthritis is most commonly due to rheumatoid arthritis, spondarthritides, osteoarthritis, chronic gout or connective tissue disease.

7. The pattern of joint involvement aids in diagnosis.
   Rheumatoid arthritis is typically symmetrical whereas spondarthritides are typically asymmetrical.

8. Joint symptoms in inflammatory conditions are characteristically worse after rest and improve with activity. Morning stiffness is a classical symptom of rheumatoid arthritis and other inflammatory arthropathies.
   Shoulder and pelvic girdle pain and stiffness which are worse in the morning may represent polymyalgia rheumatica (usually only occurs in the over 55s).

9. Patients with rheumatoid arthritis are typically unable to get moving until their joint stiffness wears off. The time taken for this is a guide to the severity of the inflammation.

11. Constant pain, especially if present at night, is a warning sign that there may be an underlying malignancy.

143

12. It is important to find out how independent the patient is at home and at work. A good way of gauging this is to ask whether they can dress themselves without assistance and whether they can walk up and down stairs without difficulty. Find out whether they have any special appliances to help them and whether they feel that they need more assistance.

13. Trauma or overuse injuries to a joint often produce swelling, stiffness and pain. Trauma, such as a fracture through a joint or repetitive injuries in sport, can predispose to osteoarthritis (then known as secondary osteoarthritis).

14. Psoriatic arthritis, reactive arthritis and SLE are all associated with skin and / or nail changes.

15. Enteropathic arthritis is an asymmetrical arthritis, predominantly affecting lower limb joints, associated with inflammatory bowel disease. The joint symptoms may pre-date the bowel disease.
    All of the spondarthritides can be associated with anterior uveitis causing eye pain and blurred vision.
    Severe rheumatoid arthritis can be associated with scleritis and episcleritis leading to painful red lesions in the eye.
    The most common cause of septic arthritis in a previously fit young adult is gonorrhoea infection.
    A reactive arthritis may follow infection with Chlamydia trachomatis. Reiter's disease is the triad of urethritis, conjunctivitis and arthritis.

16. Joints can acquire blood-borne infections from skin lesions and other sites in the body. Streptococcal pharyngitis, gonorrhoea and TB should be enquired about. Chronically inflamed joints are more prone to infection.
    Psoriasis and inflammatory bowel disease are associated with asymmetrical arthritis.
    Foot ulcers in diabetics may be complicated by osteomyelitis.
    Hypertension is a risk factor for gout as it leads to impaired secretion of uric acid.
    Osteoporosis predisposes to vertebral fractures.
    Carcinoma, myeloma and leukaemia can infiltrate the spine and lead to severe back pain.

17. All these conditions are known to have a hereditary component.

18. Find out what medications the patient has tried for their condition and whether they have experienced any side effects.
    Diuretics can precipitate gout.

19. A high alcohol intake increases serum uric acid levels so predisposes to gout. Alcohol is also a risk factor for trauma.
    Smoking is a risk factor for many malignancies.

20. Many rheumatological conditions are debilitating and severely affect people's ability to cope with everyday tasks at home and at work.

Presenting Complaint - Back Pain

		Not attempted	Attempted inadequate	Attempted adequate
1	Asks the patient to indicate the exact site of the pain	0	1	2
2	Asks whether the pain radiates anywhere else, particularly down the back of the leg.	0	1	2
3	Asks the patient whether there is any associated numbness or tingling.	0	1	2
4	Asks whether the patient has had any difficulty controlling their bladder or bowel movements.	0	1	2
5	Asks the patient when the pain began and whether the onset was sudden.	0	1	2
6	Asks whether the pain is there at rest or only on movement.	0	1	2
7	Asks whether there is anything that makes the pain better or worse.	0	1	2
8	Asks whether analgesics relieve the pain.	0	1	2
9	Asks the patient to rate the severity of the pain.	0	1	2
10	Asks whether the pain keeps the patient awake at night or wakes them up from sleep.	0	1	2
11	Asks whether the patient has strained or injured him/herself in any way recently.	0	1	2
12	Asks whether the patient has noticed any weight loss.	0	1	2
13	Asks whether the patient has had fever or night sweats.	0	1	2
14	Asks whether the patient has any bowel or eye symptoms.	0	1	2
15	Asks whether the patient has been feeling low in mood at all recently or whether they are under any particular stress at the moment.	0	1	2
16	Asks about a history of rheumatoid arthritis, osteoporosis TB or malignancies.	0	1	2

1. Musculoskeletal back pain is often well localised.
   Ankylosing spondylitis typically causes pain over the sacroiliac joints and in the buttocks.
   Pain from an osteoporotic crush fracture is usually localised to a certain vertebral level.
   The root that is affected by a prolapsed disc determines the distribution of pain.
2. Pain from a prolapsed lumbar disc radiates into the buttocks and down one leg.
   Pain from a thoracic osteoporotic crush fracture radiates around the ribs and abdomen.
   Spinal or root canal stenosis can cause buttock and bilateral leg pain.

3. Lumbar disc prolapse causes paraesthesiae and numbness, usually in one leg only. Spinal or root canal stenosis can cause bilateral paraesthesiae and numbness. Spinal cord compression causes radicular pain at the site of compression with numbness and paralysis below this level. It is a medical emergency.

4. Patients with back pain who complain of sphincter disturbance need urgent investigation as it may signify cord compression.

5. Ankylosing spondylitis usually begins in the late teenage years or early 20s. However, the diagnosis is often missed early on because the patient tends to be asymptomatic between episodes and initially, there are no radiological abnormalities. An acute disc prolapse often has a dramatic onset during a lifting, bending or twisting movement. However, it may also occur after prolonged sitting eg. in a car or aeroplane.
A crush fracture is also a sudden event usually occurring with trauma but which can sometimes be sponataneous.

6. The pain and stiffness in ankylosing spondylitis and polymyalgia rheumatica are typically worse in the morning and relieved by exercise.
Mechanical pain is aggravated by movement.
Position makes a lot of difference to mechanical back pain but not to the pain of bone disease.

7. The pain and muscular spasm of an acute disc prolapse is made worse by sitting in comparison to lying or standing.
The symptoms of spinal or root canal stenosis are relieved by rest and by bending forwards as this opens the spinal canal.

8. Pain that is not relieved by analgesics warrants further investigation.

9. This is subjective but the pain of an acute disc prolapse or a crush fracture is usually severe.
How severely the patient rates the pain may also the demonstrate the degree of effect on their lives.

10. Pain that wakes the patient from their sleep may mark an underlying malignancy.

11. The commonest cause of back pain in people aged 20-55 years is mechanical.

12. Infection or malignancy should be considered if back pain is associated with weight loss.

13. Fever or night sweats suggest infection.

14. Ankylosing spondylitis is associated with anterior uveitis and the patient may complain of eye pain and blurred vision.
Sacroilitis or spondylitis is seen in 5% of patients with inflammatory bowel disease.

15. Back pain is associated with depression.

16. Carcinoma, leukaemia and myeloma can infiltrate the spine causing unremitting back pain.
Tuberculous arthritis can affect the vertebral column leading to wedge fractures or complete vertebal collapse (Pott's disease of the spine).
Rheumatoid arthritis can affect the cervical spine.
Osteoporosis increases the risk of vertebral fractures.

Musculoskeletal Screening Examination (GALS)

		Not attempted	Attempted inadequate	Attempted adequate
1	Approaches the patient politely and introduces him/herself. Exposes the patient adequately after obtaining their permission	0	1	2
2	Asks the patient to walk, commenting on symmetry, smoothness of movement, stride length, pelvic tilt and turning instability.	0	1	2
3	Inspects the standing patient from the front, side and from behind, commenting on spinal curvature, muscle bulk and symmetry, the carrying angle of the arms and any hip or knee flexion deformity or knee hyperextension.	0	1	2
4	Places two fingers on adjacent lumbar vertebrae and asks the patient to bend forwards and touch their toes. Comments on separation of the vertebrae.	0	1	2
5	Presses over the midpoint of each supraspinatus to elicit any tenderness.	0	1	2
6	Stands in front of the patient and asks them to try to touch each shoulder in turn with the corresponding ear, commenting on cervical lateral flexion.	0	1	2
7	Asks the patient to place both hands behind their head, elbows back, commenting on any pain or restriction.	0	1	2
8	Asks the patient to place their hands behind their back and then reach as high a point as possible with their thumbs. Comments on any pain or restriction.	0	1	2
9	Asks the patient to hold both arms out, elbows locked, commenting on any fixed flexion at the elbow joint.	0	1	2
10	Asks the patient to bend their elbows so that their hands touch their shoulders.	0	1	2
11	With the elbows held flexed at 90°, asks the patient to turn their hands over, keeping their elbows in. Comments on normal supination / pronation.	0	1	2
12	Inspects the hands and wrists, commenting on any joint swelling, deformity, muscle wasting, skin / nail changes and nodules.	0	1	2
13	Squeezes across the 2nd to 5th metacarpals to elicit tenderness due to MCP synovitis.	0	1	2
14	Asks the patient to make a prayer sign with their wrists extended as far as possible. Asks them to invert this so that	0	1	2

147

	the back of their hands are in opposition with the wrists flexed.			
15	Asks them to make a tight fist with each hand, covering their nails.	0	1	2
16	Asks the patient to lie on the couch. Flexes each knee, commenting on the range of movement and any crepitus.	0	1	2
17	Internally and externally rotates each hip in flexion commenting on any pain or restriction.	0	1	2
18	Tests for any effusion over the knee using the bulge sign and the patellar tap.	0	1	2
19	Squeezes across the metatarsals for any tenderness.	0	1	2
20	Inspects both soles for any calluses reflecting abnormal weight bearing.	0	1	2
21	Thanks patient and washes hands			

1. It is important to introduce yourself (give your name and what you do) and explain that would like to examine their muscles and joints. Explain that you need to expose them fully in order to perform an adequate examination. Respect the modesty of patients. Explain what you are going to do as you proceed with the examination, *before* you do it!
2. Try and decide whether the gait fits any recognised pathological pattern (see examination of the neurological system). Does the gait appear painful?
3. Look for asymmetry and try to assess the overall pattern of visible joint involvement. A normal spine should have a cervical lordosis, a thoracic kyphosis and a lumbar lordosis. Loss of the lumbar lordosis is characteristic of ankylosing spondylitis. Scoliosis can result from developmental abnormalities, trauma, muscle disease or vertebral body disease.
   The normal elbow has a carrying angle of 5-10° valgus. This is increased in Turner's syndrome.
   At the knees, look particularly for varus, valgus, flexion deformities and Baker's cysts.
   At the feet, look particularly for hallux valgus, hindfoot valgus, toe crowding and flattened arches which can all occur as part of rheumatoid arthritis.
   Muscles acting at diseased joints often waste through disuse.
4. Serial assessment of lumbar flexion can give an idea of disease progression.
5. This is one of the recognised tender points of fibromyalgia.
6. Lateral flexion is normally possible to 45° (although decreases with age). It is the most sensitive movement to symptomatic lesions.
7. This tests shoulder abduction and external rotation, important movements for reaching out and for combing hair.
   Abduction to 90° occurs at the glenohumoral joint. Further elevation involves the scapulothoracic joint.
8. This tests internal rotation at the shoulder joint, an important movement for dressing and washing.
9. Inability to fully extend the elbows occurs in synovitis, osteoarthritis, soft tissue conditions and trauma.
10. The elbow should flex to 150°.
11. These are important functional movements. It is important that the arms are adducted during this test because pronation can otherwise be achieved using the shoulder joint.

12. Look for loss of joint contours as a marker of swelling.

Synovitis may be visible as swellings around joints or swelling of the tendon sheaths. Deformity can be due to damage to the joint or surrounding soft tissue or to tendon rupture.

Ulnar deviation of the phalanges and MCP joints, swan neck and boutonniere deformities of the fingers and Z deformity of the thumb are characteristic findings in rheumatoid arthritis.

Osteoarthritis usually affects the DIP and 1st carpometacarpal joints (leading to squaring of the base of the thumb). Osteophytes are often present and known as Heberden's nodes at the DIP joints and Bouchard's nodes at the PIP joints.

Sausage shaped fingers are characteristic of psoriatic arthritis but also occur in Reiter's disease.

Contraction deformities of the fingers are common in scleroderma.

Always note the symmetry of any joint involvement.

13. Tenderness across the joints suggests that there is inflammation present. In this case, go on to feel each joint individually for synovial thickening.
14. This is a good test to see if there is any fixed flexion of the MCP and IP joints. It also tests flexion and extension at the wrists (are the arms at the same level?) and allows symmetry of the hands to be assessed.
15. They should be able to make a fist such that their palm covers their nails.
16. Knee flexion should be limited by the calf touching the thigh.
Crepitus is produced when there are loose bodies within the joint or when the articular surfaces are irregular, as occurs in osteoarthritis.
17. Moving the foot laterally results in internal rotation of the hip.
The range of movement of internal rotation is smaller than for external rotation so internal rotation is the more sensitive marker of abnormality.
18. There are several ways of detecting effusions including visible loss of the concavities on either side of the patella, the bulge sign and the patella tap.
The bulge sign is used to detect small effusions. Empty any fluid from one side of the knee to the other by sliding the flat of your hand along the side of the knee. Then transfer your hand to the opposite side of the knee and run the back of the hand along in a similar manner, looking for a bulge appearing on the side you first emptied.
To test for larger effusions, empty the supra-patella pouch by straddling the thigh with your open hand, thumb and forefingers on either side of the thigh in order to lift the patella clear of the femur. Then steady your examining hand by placing your fingertips on the tibia so that your thumb comes down in the middle of the patella to ascertain if a "tap" can be felt as the patella comes back into contact with the femur.
19. Tenderness of the joints occurs in inflammatory conditions but also in conditions that are regarded conventionally as being non-inflammatory such as osteoarthritis.
20. Subluxation of the metatarsal heads predisposes to callus formation.
21. It is polite to thank the patient. Always wash your hands to reduce the risk of cross-infection.

Examination Of The Hands

		Not attempted	Attempted inadequate	Attempted adequate
1	Approaches the patient politely and introduces him/herself. Exposes the patient adequately (to above the elbows on both sides) after obtaining their permission.	0	1	2
2	Inspects the dorsum of the hand and wrist, comparing it to the other side and commenting on the overlying skin, any muscle wasting and any swelling or deformity.	0	1	2
3	Inspects the nails, commenting on any changes.	0	1	2
4	Inspects the palmar surfaces of the hands commenting on any scars, muscle wasting or erythema.	0	1	2
5	Asks the patient to flex their fingers whilst the examiner palpates over the flexor tendons in the palm.	0	1	2
6	Palpates the anatomical snuff box for tenderness.	0	1	2
7	Palpates the wrist, MCP, PIP and DIP joints commenting on any tenderness, swelling and the nature of the swelling.	0	1	2
8	Asks the patient to make as tight a fist as possible.	0	1	2
9	Asks the patient to make the prayer sign and then the inverted prayer sign.	0	1	2
10	Tests the motor divisions of the radial, ulnar and median nerves.	0	1	2
11	Tests the sensory divisions of the radial, ulnar and median nerves.	0	1	2
12	Taps over the flexor retinaculum to test for Tinel's sign.	0	1	2
13	Palpates the radial pulse.			
14	Inspects the elbows for rheumatoid nodules or gouty tophi.			
15	Tests function of the hands by asking the patient to fasten a button, grip a pen etc.			
16	Thanks patient and washes hands			

1. It is important to introduce yourself (give your name and what you do) and explain that you would like to examine their hands. Explain what you are going to do as you proceed with the examination, *before* you do it!

2. See point 12 of examination of the musculoskeletal system.

3. Pitting, onycholysis, hyperkeratosis, ridging and discolouration of the nails can all occur as features of psoriasis.

Splinter haemorrhages can be due to vasculitis occurring as part of rheumatoid arthritis or SLE. However, they can also be due to trauma to the nail.

4. Scars on the palms may be from tendon replacement operations.
    Muscle wasting through disuse, vasculitis or peripheral nerve entrapment may be evident at the thenar or hypothenar eminences where it leads to loss of convexity.

5. Palmar tendon crepitus will be felt if there is tenosynovitis (the inflamed tendons creak in their thickened sheaths and nodules may be palpable).
    Nodules may become sufficiently large to stick in a narrowing of the tendon sheath causing a flexion deformity from which the finger can only be extended by force. This is a trigger finger and can occur in rheumatoid arthritis.

6. This will be tender in fractures of the scaphoid.

7. Palpation of the joints should be done in sets eg. MCPs, PIPs etc. Palpate in two planes: anteroposterior for tenderness and laterally for synovitis or bony swelling. Osteophytes that were missed on inspection might be picked up on palpation. Dorsal subluxation of the ulnar head due to laxity of the ligaments supporting the distal radioulnar joint is a characteristic feature of rheumatoid arthritis.

8. See point 15 of examination of the musculoskeletal system.

9. See point 14 of examination of the musculoskeletal system.

10. Ask the patient to cock their wrists and resist you pushing them down (radial nerve), abduct their thumb and resist you pushing it down (median nerve) and abduct their fingers and resist you pushing them together (ulnar nerve).

11. Tests whether the patient can detect touch over the base of the thumb (radial nerve), the medial border of the hand (ulnar nerve) and the lateral border of the index finger (median nerve). It is important to compare sensation on the medial and lateral borders of the hand.

12. Tinel's sign is positive if tapping over the flexor retinaculum leads to paraesthesiae in the distribution of the median nerve. It indicates that the flexor retinaculum is thickened and has trapped the nerve in the carpal tunnel.

13. It is important to check the adequacy of the circulation, especially if surgery may be required.

14. The elbows are a common site for rheumatoid nodules and gouty tophi which can aid in the diagnosis of signs already picked up in the hands.

15. This allows composite movement to be assessed.
16. It is polite to thank the patient. Always wash your hands to reduce the risk of cross-infection.

Examination Of The Hip

		Not attempted	Attempted inadequate	Attempted adequate
1	Approaches the patient politely and introduces him/herself. Exposes the patient adequately after obtaining their permission.	0	1	2
2	Inspects the hips and legs commenting on scars, swelling, skin abnormalities, deformity and muscle wasting.	0	1	2
3	Inspects the patient from the end of the bed, commenting on any discrepancy in leg length.	0	1	2
4	Feels for tenderness over the greater trochanter, the iliac crest and in the groin.	0	1	2
5	Flexes the hips, one at a time, commenting on range of movement and any fixed flexion deformity that becomes apparent.	0	1	2
6	Externally and internally rotates the hip joints whilst they are still flexed, commenting on range of movement.	0	1	2
7	Abducts and adducts the hip joints with the leg extended, commenting on range of movement.	0	1	2
8	Asks the patient to roll onto their front, if they are able, and tests hip extension.	0	1	2
9	Asks the patient to turn back and feels for dorsalis pedis and posterior tibial pulses.	0	1	2
10	Tests sensation over the legs.	0	1	2
11	Tests active movements of the feet and ankle joints.	0	1	2
12	Asks the patient to stand and comments on any deformity that becomes apparent.	0	1	2
13	Performs Trendelenburg's test.	0	1	2
14	Asks the patient to walk, commenting on the gait.	0	1	2
15	Thanks patient and washes hands.			

1. It is important to introduce yourself (give your name and what you do) and explain that you would like to examine their hip joints. Explain that you need to expose them fully in order to perform an adequate examination. Respect the modesty of patients. Explain what you are going to do as you proceed with the examination, *before* you do it!

2. A scar from a hip replacement is on the lateral aspect of the hip.
   Signs of infection should always be looked for, as infection is a contraindication to any orthopaedic surgery.
   Swelling of the hip joint is rarely visible.

A dislocated hip causes the leg to be held adducted and flexed.

A fractured neck of femur often causes the leg to be shortened and externally rotated.

A painful hip with synovitis is most comfortable if held in slight flexion, abduction and external rotation.

3. True leg length is measured from the anterior superior iliac spine to the medial malleolus. Any difference in this indicates hip disease on the shorter side or a previous fracture.

   Apparent leg length is measured from the umbilicus to the medial malleolus. Discrepancies in this are either due to true shortening or to tilting of the pelvis.

4. These are the three sites of likely tenderness if there is hip pathology.

   Tenderness over the greater trochanter may be due to trochanteric bursitis.

5. Normal hip flexion is limited by the knee touching the chest.

   Thomas' test for fixed flexion deformity of the hip involves placing your hand under the patient's lumbar spine whilst flexing their hip. As the lumbar lordosis flattens out, any fixed flexion in the other hip becomes apparent.

6. Normal hips have 45° of external rotation and 35° of internal rotation.

7. Normal hips have 40° of abduction and 20° of adduction.

   Whilst performing these movements, place your hand over the contralateral anterior superior iliac spine. The pelvis will be felt to move at the limit of abduction.

8. When testing hip extension, place one hand over the sacroiliac joint and use the other to elevate the leg. It's normally possible to get about 10° of movement.

9. The circulation below the diseased joint should always be checked especially if the patient is likely to need surgery. If dorsalis pedis and posterior tibial pulses are impalpable, more proximal pulses should be felt for to assess the level of the deficit.

10. It is important to document any sensory deficit present before surgery.

11. Asking the patient to actively move their feet and ankles is sufficient to check that the motor system in the lower legs is grossly intact but a formal neurological assessment of the motor system may be necessary.

12. Compensation for shortening of one leg is achieved by scoliotic posture or flexion of the longer leg.

    Flexion deformity is compensated for by an exaggerated lordosis.

13. Trendelenburg's test assesses the integrity of the hip abductors.

    Observing from behind, ask the patient to stand on one leg. If the muscles are functioning correctly, the pelvis will rise on the non-weight bearing side and balance will be maintained. If the muscles are weak, as in an L5 root lesion, proximal myopathy or hip joint disease, the non-weight bearing side will sag.

14. Look particularly for a limp or a waddling gait (which occurs if Trendelenburg's test is positive bilaterally).

15. It is polite to thank the patient. Always wash your hands to reduce the risk of cross-infection.

Examination Of The Knee

		Not attempted	Attempted inadequate	Attempted adequate
1	Approaches the patient politely and introduces him/herself. Exposes the patient adequately after obtaining their permission.	0	1	2
2	Inspects the knees commenting on scars, swelling, erythema, deformity and muscle wasting.	0	1	2
3	Feels for tenderness over the joint line with the knee in flexion and then on patella movement with the knee extended. Comments on the warmth of the skin over the knee joints and on any crepitus.	0	1	2
4	Feels for an effusion using the bulge sign and the patella tap test.	0	1	2
5	Flexes the knees, one at a time, commenting on range of movement.	0	1	2
6	Checks that the knees are capable of full extension.	0	1	2
7	Looks for evidence of a posterior cruciate ligament rupture by looking from the side at the patient's flexed knees.	0	1	2
8	Performs the anterior draw test and Lachman's test to test for an anterior cruciate ligament rupture.	0	1	2
9	Assesses the integrity of the medial and lateral collateral ligaments.	0	1	2
10	Assess the stability of the menisci using McMurray's test.	0	1	2
11	Feels for dorsalis pedis and posterior tibial pulses.	0	1	2
12	Tests sensation over the legs.	0	1	2
13	Tests active movements of the feet and ankle joints.	0	1	2
14	Asks the patient to walk, commenting on the gait.	0	1	2
15	Thanks patient and washes hands			

1. It is important to introduce yourself (give your name and what you do) and explain that you would like to examine their knee. Explain that you need to expose them fully in order to perform an adequate examination but always respect their modesty. Explain what you are going to do as you proceed with the examination, *before* you do it!

2. Valgus and varus deformities are best assessed with the patient standing. Large effusions may be visible but smaller ones will only be detectable by palpation. Osteoarthritis of the knee leads to bony swelling and wasting of the quadriceps.

3. The knee needs to be slightly flexed to enable the joint line to be palpated. This will be tender in osteoarthritis of the knee and if there is meniscal injury.
    A patient with recurrent dislocation of the patella will not like their patella being moved laterally. Feel in the popliteal fossa for a Baker's cyst.

4. See point 18 of the general musculoskeletal examination.

5. Knee flexion should be limited by the calf touching the thigh.

6. Stand at the foot of the bed and lift both of the patient's legs slightly off the bed. The knees will fall into full extension if there is no limitation to movement. Typically a tear in the medial meniscus causes the knee to lock, preventing full extension. An anterior cruciate ligament tear or bony swelling in osteoarthritis can also prevent full extension.

7. With the patient's feet flat on the bed so that the knees are flexed to 90°, the tibias should be at the same level. If one is sagging back, it indicates that the posterior cruciate ligament is damaged.

8. To carry out the anterior draw test, ask the patient to keep their knees bent to 90° whilst you sit on their foot to stabilise the leg (providing this does not cause them pain). Pull forwards on the knee joint, keeping your thumbs on the tibia, to see if there is abnormal movement indicating an anterior cruciate ligament tear. Lachman's test is also used to assess the anterior cruciate ligament. It is more sensitive than the anterior draw test. Place your knee on the bed so that it supports the patient's knee in 30° of flexion. Steady the thigh with one hand and pull forwards on the upper calf with the other hand. Laxity indicates a torn anterior cruciate ligament.

9. To assess the collateral ligaments, sit on the bed and support the patient's leg so that their foot is held in your axilla and their knee is slightly flexed. Stress the collaterals in both directions by attempting to abduct and adduct the lower leg with one hand holding above the knee and one below.

10. To carry out McMurray's test, hold the patient's heel with your right hand so that their hip and knee are flexed to 90°. Steady the knee with your left hand and slowly extend the knee, first with the tibia in external rotation and then in internal rotation. If the meniscus is unstable it will displace with a 'clunk' and the patient will experience some discomfort.

11-13. See points 9, 10 and 11 of the hip examination.

14. Look for an antalgic gait.
15. It is polite to thank the patient. Always wash your hands to reduce the risk of cross-infection.

Examination Of A Patient With Back Pain

		Not attempted	Attempted inadequate	Attempted adequate
1	Approaches the patient politely and introduces him/herself. Exposes the patient adequately after obtaining their permission.	0	1	2
2	Inspects the patient with them standing, from the side and from behind, commenting on spinal curvature and symmetry.	0	1	2
3	Asks the patient to bend forwards, backwards and sideways, commenting on range of movement.	0	1	2
4	Palpates for tenderness over the spinous processes and the paraspinal muscles.	0	1	2
5	Asks the patient to walk a few steps on tiptoes and then on their heels.	0	1	2
6	Asks the patient to lie on his/her back and performs the straight leg raise test. If there is pain, repeats the movement with the knee flexed.	0	1	2
7	Tests power in the lower limbs, comparing both sides.	0	1	2
8	Tests the reflexes in both lower limbs, comparing sides.	0	1	2
9	Tests sensation in the lower limb, comparing both sides.	0	1	2
10	Asks the patient to turn so that they are lying prone and asks them to clench their buttocks.	0	1	2
11	Tests sensation over the buttocks and perineum.	0	1	2
12	Goes on to examine the breasts, thyroid, abdomen and lymph nodes if the history suggests that it is applicable.	0	1	2
13	Thanks patient and washes hands			

1. It is important to introduce yourself (give your name and what you do) and explain that you would like to examine them . Explain that you need to expose them fully in order to perform an adequate examination. Respect the modesty of patients. Explain what you are going to do as you proceed with the examination, *before* you do it!

2. Scoliosis is defined by the level of the spine and the side of the convexity of the curve. It may be postural (will correct on forward flexion) or structural.
An increased thoracic kyphosis may be smooth due to multilevel disease or sharply angulated due to local vertebral destruction.
A patient with pain due to a prolapsed lumbar disc will often stand with their knees slighly flexed to relieve root compression.

3. Forward flexion comes from spinal movement and hip flexion. To assess the vertebral movement, place two fingers on adjacent vertebrae and note the degree of separation of the fingers as the patient bends forward.

Extension may be particularly painful with facet joint damage.
If sideways flexion is more limited than forward flexion, it suggests ankylosing spondylitis.

4. Local tenderness confirms that the pain arises from the back rather than being referred pain eg. from a pelvic organ.
   Any steps in the alignment of the interspinous processes may represent a spondylolisthesis.

5. An S1 root lesion will make walking on the toes difficult whereas an L4/5 root lesion will make walking on the heels difficult (due to footdrop).

6. Place one hand on the pelvis and the other under the ankle. Elevate the straight leg whilst watching the patient's face for distress.
   The normal range of movement is 70°. This can be limited by a stiff hip as well as by an irritated sciatic nerve. However, with sciatica, the hips should flex painlessly if the knee is bent.

7. Weak quadriceps suggest L4 root damage.
   Weakness of the muscles of the foot and ankle suggest L5 root damage (weak tibialis anterior and extensor hallucis longus).
   S1 root damage causes weakness of soleus.

8. S1 root compression leads to loss of the ankle jerk reflex.
   L4 root compression leads to loss of the knee jerk reflex.

9. A sensory deficit in a dermatomal distribution suggests nerve root compression.

10. One buttock failing to clench as much as the other is a sign of neurological damage.

11. Anaesthesia around the anus or loss of the anal wink reflex (contraction of the external sphincter in response to scratching the perianal skin) are associated with cauda equina lesions and need urgent investigation.

12. If the patient looks ill or has given a history of weight loss or night sweats with unremitting pain, a general examination is particularly necessary.

13. It is polite to thank the patient. Always wash your hands to reduce the risk of cross-infection.

Rheumatic fever: Revised Jones' criteria

JONES PEACE:
· Major criteria:
Joints: migratory
O (heart shaped) Carditis: new onset murmur
Nodules, subcutaneous: extensor surfaces
Erythema marginatum
Sydenham's chorea
· Minor criteria:
PR interval, prolonged
ESR elevated
Arthralgias
CRP elevated
Elevated temperature (fever)
· Need 2 major or 1 major and 2 minor criteria, plus evidence of recent GAS infection (throat cx, rapid antigen test, or rising strep antibody titer).

Side effects of steroids

BECLOMETHASONE
Buffalo hump
Easy bruising
Cataracts
Larger appetite
Obesity
Moonface
Euphoria
Thin arms & legs
Hypertension/ **H**yperglycaemia
Avascular necrosis of femoral head
Skin thinning
Osteoporosis
Negative nitrogen balance
Emotional liability

The Endocrine System

General Endocrine History

		Not attempted	Attempted inadequate	Attempted adequate
1	Approaches the patient politely and introduces him/herself.	0	1	2
2	Asks the patient's name, DOB and occupation.	0	1	2
3	Asks about history of appetite and weight changes.	0	1	2
4	Asks about history of altered bowel habit.	0	1	2
5	Asks about her menstrual and obstetric histories.	0	1	2
6	Asks about history of impotence.	0	1	2
7	Asks about history of excessive sweating.	0	1	2
8	Asks about history of change in hair distribution.	0	1	2
9	Asks about history of lethargy.	0	1	2
10	Asks about history of skin changes.	0	1	2
11	Asks about history of a lump in the neck.	0	1	2
12	Asks whether the patient has been passing more urine recently or whether they have felt unusually thirsty.	0	1	2
13	Asks about history of headache or visual disturbance.	0	1	2
14	Asks how the patient has been feeling mentally and emotionally.	0	1	2
15	Asks about relevant past or current conditions including thyroid disease, hypertension, diabetes, pituitary disease and TB.	0	1	2
16	Asks about family history of thyroid conditions, diabetes mellitus, pituitary tumours, phaeochromocytoma and pancreatic tumours.	0	1	2
17	Asks about smoking and alcohol consumption.	0	1	2
18	Asks about home and work circumstances.	0	1	2
19	Asks about past and current medications and any allergies to medication.	0	1	2

1. It is polite to introduce yourself and explain your task.

2. Name: to establish rapport and identify the patient.
   Age/DOB: certain diseases affect certain age groups e.g. type I DM usually presents in childhood whereas type II usually has a later onset. The DOB should be recorded to identify the patient.
   Occupation: this provides information about the patient's background and can have significant effects on the management of their condition. Jobs which involve exposure to radiation may be of relevance in the aetiology of thyroid disorders.

3. Increased appetite with weight loss classically occurs in thyrotoxicosis or in uncontrolled DM.
   Increased appetite with weight gain occurs in Cushing's syndrome.
   Loss of appetite with weight loss can occur in adrenal insufficiency (but is also seen in GI disease).
   Weight gain often occurs in hypothyroidism.

4. Hyperthyroidism can cause diarrhoea.
   Hypothyroidism and hypercalcaemia can cause constipation.

5. Primary amenorrhoea can be due to gonadal dysgenesis, anatomical abnormalities or testicular feminisation.
   The differential for secondary amenorrhoea is extremely large. It can be caused by a problem anywhere in the axis from the pituitary to the uterus. Common causes include excessive exercise or weight loss, medications, thyroid dysfunction, pituitary tumours, ovarian failure, PCOS and pregnancy.
   The menopause can be a cause of increased sweating, menstrual irregularities (in the few months leading up to the menopause) and emotional disturbance.
   Gestational diabetes should be enquired about as women who have had this are at a higher risk of developing diabetes in later life.

6. Physical causes of impotence include neuropathies (e.g. DM), hypertension, vascular disease, alcohol, recreational drugs and side effects of anti-hypertensives, anti-depressants and steroids.

7. Hyperthyroidism, phaeochromocytoma, hypoglycaemia and acromegaly all lead to increased sweating.

8. Hirsutism and temporal recession of scalp hair in women occur in conditions of androgen excess including PCOS, Cushing's syndrome and acromegaly.
   Absence of facial hair in men suggests hypogonadism.
   Loss of axillary or pubic hair in females suggests adrenal insufficiency but in males it suggests hypopituitarism (loss of adrenal and testicular androgen secretion).

9. Lethargy occurs in hypothyroidism, Addison's disease and DM but also occurs in many other diseases and is a side effect of many drugs.

10. Hypothyroidism causes the skin to become coarse, pale and dry.
    Acromegaly, diabetes, Cushing's syndrome and PCOS are all associated with acanthosis nigricans (pigmented papillomatous growths, mainly in the armpits).
    An excess of glucocorticoids leads to atrophy of the skin, associated with easy bruising and striae.
    Primary hypoadrenalism leads to compensatory ACTH hypersecretion and these patients may therefore notice pigmentation in the palmar creases, elbows, gums and

buccal mucosa and in any scars. Patients with Cushing's disease (pituitary ACTH over-production) may also get increased pigmentation.

11. Most lumps in the neck are enlarged lymph nodes but the patient may notice a goitre, which can be associated with thyroid dysfunction.

12. Polyuria can occur in DM, diabetes insipidus and hypercalcaemia. Primary polydipsia, which is usually psychogenic in origin, can also cause polyuria.

13. Pituitary adenomas classically cause a bitemporal hemianopia as they compress the optic chiasm. They can also press on the bony structures and meninges surrounding the pituitary fossa.

14. Many endocrine conditions can lead to psychological disturbance.
Cushing's syndrome, hypothyroidism, DM and adrenocortical insufficiency can lead to depression.
Thyrotoxicosis, hypothyroidism, hypoparathyrodism, phaeochromocytoma and hypoglycaemia can lead to delirium.
Hypothyroidism can cause dementia.
Anxiety and panic disorder can be caused by hyperthyroidism, phaeochromocytoma and hypoparathyroidism.

15. The presence of one organ-specific autoimmune disease increases the chances of developing another.
Treatment for thyrotoxicosis may lead to hypothyroidism. Thyroid surgery may damage the parathyroid glands and so be associated with hypoparathyroidism.
Hypertension may have an endocrine cause such as Cushing's syndrome, acromegaly or Conn's syndrome.
TB can be a cause of primary adrenal failure.

16. Organ-specific autoimmune diseases have a strong hereditary component. Pituitary tumours, medullary carcinoma of the thyroid, hyperparathyroidism, phaeochromocytoma and pancreatic tumours may all be part of the multiple endocrine neoplasia (MEN) syndrome (an autosomal dominant condition).

17. Alcohol can precipitate a hypoglycaemic episode in diabetics. It can also lead to a pseudo-cushing's syndrome.
Smoking in conjunction with DM and hypertension will further increase the risk of cardiovascular disease.
Smoking also predisposes to small cell carcinoma of the lung, which can be a source of ectopic ACTH.

18. Many endocrine conditions are chronic and have serious complications. The patient's home and work environment will have an important impact on how they cope and how they respond to treatment.

19. The commonest cause of Cushing's disease is excess exogenous administration of steroids.
Abrupt cessation of prolonged high-dose corticosteroid therapy can lead to acute adrenocortical insufficiency.
Lithium and amiodarone can lead to hypothyroidism. Amiodarone can also lead to thyrotoxicosis.

Symptoms of Acromegaly

ABCDEF:
Arthralgia/ **A**rthritis
Blood pressure raised
Carpal tunnel syndrome
Diabetes
Enlarged organs
Field defect

Symptoms of SIADH

SIADH:
Spasms
Isn't any pitting edema (key DDx)
Anorexia
Disorientation (and other psychoses)
Hyponatremia

Causes of SIADH

SIADH:
Surgery
Intracranial: infection, head injury, CVA
Alveolar: Ca, pus
Drugs: opiates,antiepileptics, cytotoxics, anti-psychotics
Hormonal: hypothyroid, low corticosteroid level

Suspected Diabetes Mellitus

		Not attempted	Attempted inadequate	Attempted adequate
1	Asks the patient how many times a day they have to pass water on average.	0	1	2
2	Asks whether the patient gets unusually thirsty.	0	1	2
3	Asks the patient whether they have noticed any change in weight recently.	0	1	2
4	Asks whether the patient feels unusually tired or lethargic.	0	1	2
5	Asks whether the patient has any problems with their eyesight.	0	1	2
6	Asks whether the patient regularly suffers from infections.	0	1	2
7	Asks whether the patient has noticed any tingling or numbness in their hands or feet.	0	1	2
8	Asks whether the patient suffers from impotence.	0	1	2
9	Asks about history of heart disease or strokes.	0	1	2
10	Asks if the patient is on any medications, specifically steroids.	0	1	2
11	Asks the patient how much alcohol they drink.	0	1	2
12	Asks whether there is any family history of diabetes.			

1. Polyuria in DM is due to an osmotic diuresis secondary to glycosuria.
   Diabetes insipidus also leads to polyuria as the deficiency of, or insensivity to, ADH leads to inadequate renal water conservation.

2. Hypertonicity of the extracellular fluid, due to the osmotic diuresis, leads to an increased perception of thirst.

3. Recent weight loss can be evidence of uncontrolled glycosuria.
   Many patients who develop type II DM are chronically obese.

4. Patients with uncontrolled DM can present with lethargy and tiredness.

5. Visual disturbances in diabetes can be due to retinal vascular disease or due to changes in the shape of the lens associated with hyperglycaemia and water retention.

6. Skin infections are common in diabetics because the combination of high tissue glucose levels and ischaemia provides a favourable environment for the growth of organisms.
   Poorly controlled diabetes increases susceptibility to urinary tract and respiratory infections.

7. Diabetic neuropathy can be a presenting feature in older patients with diabetes who may have had unrecognised disease for months or years. Symptoms are usually in

the feet with involvement of the hands being much less common (glove and stocking distribution).

8. Impotence can be due to autonomic neuropathy secondary to diabetes but there are many other psychological and physiological causes that need to be considered.

9. Diabetes is a risk factor for atherosclerosis.

10. Corticosteroid excess leads to hyperglycaemia and in some cases, diabetes.

11. Alcoholics are at risk of developing chronic pancreatitis complicated by DM. Diabetics need to be warned that alcohol induces hypoglycaemia as it inhibits gluconeogenesis.

12. There is some degree of genetic susceptibility for both type I and type II DM.

Suspected Thyroid Dysfunction

		Not attempted	Attempted inadequate	Attempted adequate
1	Asks the patient whether they have noticed any change in their appetite or weight recently.	0	1	2
2	Asks the patient whether they prefer warm or cool environments.	0	1	2
3	Asks whether the patient feels that they sweat more than other people or if they have noticed themselves sweating more recently.	0	1	2
4	Asks the patient if their bowel habit has changed recently.	0	1	2
5	Asks whether the patient ever gets an awareness of their heart beating.	0	1	2
6	Asks whether the patient feels unusually nervous or irritable.	0	1	2
7	Asks the patient if her periods are regular and whether they are particularly heavy.	0	1	2
8	Asks the patient if they get breathless on exertion.	0	1	2
9	Asks whether they suffer from muscle weakness.	0	1	2
10	Asks whether the patient has noticed a tremor of their hands.	0	1	2
11	Asks whether the patient feels unusually lethargic.	0	1	2
12	Asks the patient whether they have developed any problems with their eyes.	0	1	2
13	Asks whether the patient has noticed any change in character of their voice.	0	1	2
14	Asks whether they feel their skin is particularly coarse.	0	1	2
15	Asks whether they have noticed a lump in their neck.	0	1	2
16	Asks whether they have a family history of thyroid dysfunction.	0	1	2
17	Asks whether they take any medications.	0	1	2

1. Thyrotoxicosis leads to an increased appetite with weight loss.
   Hypothyroidism typically leads to weight gain.

2. Thyrotoxicosis is associated with a preference for cool conditions whereas hypothyroidism is associated with a preference for warm environments.

3. Increased sweating is characteristic of hyperthyroidism.

4. Hyperthyroidism may be associated with diarrhoea.
   Hypothyroidism may be associated with constipation.

5. Thyrotoxicosis can induce palpitations.

6. Nervousness and irritability are characteristic of thyrotoxicosis.

7. Hypo or hyperthyroidism can both lead to menstrual changes.

8. Thyrotoxicosis is often associated with breathlessness especially if there is a tachycardia or cardiac arrhythmia.
   A retrosternal goitre may cause thoracic inlet obstruction leading to respiratory distress and stridor when the arms are raised above the head (Pemberton's sign).

9. Proximal myopathy can occur with thyrotoxicosis or hypothyroidism.

10. A fine tremor is a sign of thyrotoxicosis.

11. Lethargy is associated with hypothyroidism.

12. Periorbital oedema occurs in hypothyroidism.
    In Grave's disease, problems with the eyes such as double vision, proptosis and periorbital oedema may occur and require urgent attention.

13. Coarse, croaking slow speech is typical of hypothyroidism.

14. In severe hypothyroidism, myxoedema can occur with accumulation of hydrophilic mucopolysaccharides in the skin leading to thickening and a doughy induration.

15. The patient may notice a goitre, which can be associated with thyroid dysfunction.

16. Autoimmune thyroid conditions have a strong genetic component.

17. Lithium and amiodarone can both disturb thyroid function.

Examination For Hypothyroidism

		Not attempted	Attempted inadequate	Attempted adequate
1	Approaches the patient politely and introduces him/herself. Exposes the patient adequately after obtaining their permission.	0'	1	2
2	Performs a general inspection looking for dry skin, obesity and periorbital oedema.	0	1	2
3	Looks at and feels the hands commenting on swelling of the skin, temperature and dryness.	0	1	2
4	Feels the radial pulse commenting on rate, rhythm and volume.	0	1	2
5	Taps over the flexor retinaculum to test for carpal tunnel thickening.	0	1	2
6	Inspects the face commenting on the appearance of the skin, alopecia areata and vitiligo and feels for dryness and coolness of the skin and hair.	0	1	2
7	Examines for a goitre.	0	1	2
8	Tests the power and reflexes in the patient's arms and legs.	0	1	2
9	Thanks patient and washes hands	0	1	2

1. It is important to introduce yourself (give your name and what you do) and explain that you would like to examine them. Explain that you need to expose them fully in order to perform an adequate examination. Respect the modesty of patients. Explain what you are going to do as you proceed with the examination, *before* you do it!
2. This is the characteristic appearance of a patient with hypothyroidism.
   Also take note of whether the patient is dressed appropriately for the conditions - a hypothyroid patient may be wearing warmer clothes than the average person would require.
3. The skin may be swollen due to the accumulation of mucopolysaccharides and interstitial fluid, and is typically cool and dry.
4. The pulse will typically be small volume and slow in hypothyroidism.
5. If the flexor retinaculum is thickened by myxoedema it may entrap the median nerve in the carpal tunnel. Tapping over the retinaculum will lead to paraesthesiae in the nerve's distribution (Tinel's sign).
6. The skin and hair will be cool, dry and coarse.
   Vitiligo and alopecia areata are autoimmune diseases which may be associated with autoimmune thyroid disease.
   Loss of hair, particularly the outer third of the eyebrows, can be a feature of hypothyroidism.
7. See the section on examination of a goitre.
   Causes of hypothyroidism associated with an enlarged gland include iodine deficiency, Hashimoto's thyroiditis or drug effects e.g. amiodarone.
8. See the neurological examination sections for how to perform these.
   Proximal myopathy can occur in hypothyroidism but is rare.
   Hypothyroidism leads to 'hung up' reflexes in which a normal contraction is followed by delayed relaxation.

Examination For Thyrotoxicosis

		Not attempted	Attempted inadequate	Attempted adequate
1	Approaches the patient politely and introduces him/herself. Exposes the patient adequately after obtaining their permission.	0	1	2
2	Performs a general inspection commenting on tremor, sweating and signs of anxiety.	0	1	2
3	Looks at the hands commenting on onycholysis, thyroid acropachy and palmar erythema.	0	1	2
4	Feels the rate and rhythm of the radial pulse and tests for a collapsing pulse.	0	1	2
5	Asks the patient to hold their hands out in front of them and comments on any tremor evident.	0	1	2
6	Inspects the eyes commenting on lid retraction, proptosis, conjunctivitis and corneal ulceration.	0	1	2
7	Tests the eye movements commenting on any ophthalmoplegia.	0	1	2
8	Tests for lid lag by asking the patient to follow a finger with their eyes as it descends at a moderate rate from the upper to lower part of the visual field.	0	1	2
9	Examines for a goitre.	0	1	2
10	Inspects the legs for pretibial myxoedema.	0	1	2
11	Tests power and reflexes in the legs and arms.	0	1	2
12	Auscultates the heart for systolic flow murmurs.	0	1	2
13	Thanks patient and washes hands	0	1	2

1. It is important to introduce yourself (give your name and what you do) and explain that you would like to examine them. Explain that you need to expose them fully in order to perform an adequate examination. Respect the modesty of patients. Explain what you are going to do as you proceed with the examination, *before* you do it!

2. Sweating, tremor and anxiety are manifestations of sympathetic overactivity and are typical of thyrotoxicosis.

3. Onycholysis is separation of the nail from its bed and thyroid acropachy is clubbing. Both of these are rare features of Grave's disease. Palmar erythema can occur in thyrotoxicosis of any cause.

4. Sinus tachycardia and atrial fibrillation are both common findings in thyrotoxicosis. The high cardiac output may result in a collapsing pulse.

5. Thyrotoxicosis is associated with a fine tremor.

6. Proptosis is protrusion of the eyeball out of the orbit. Mild forms may be recognised by the fact that the sclerae are not covered by the lower lid and eye is visible anterior to the superior orbital margin when inspected from over the patient's forehead. It is only seen in Grave's disease.
   Conjunctivitis may be a complication of proptosis.
   Corneal ulceration may occur when there is inability to close the eyelids.

7. Ophthalmoplegia may also be found in Grave's disease, probably due to inflammatory infiltrate of the orbital muscles.

8. If lid lag is present, descent of the upper lid lags behind descent of the gaze. This sign is related to sympathetic overactivity and is not specific for Grave's disease.

9. See the section on examination of a goitre.
   Causes of a goitre in thyrotoxic patients include Grave's disease, toxic multinodular goitre, toxic adenoma or DeQuervain's thyroiditis.
   Thyrotoxicosis can also occur without a goitre, particularly in the elderly.

10. Pretibial myxoedema is seen as bilateral firm elevated dermal nodules and plaques occurring over the shins. It is a feature of Grave's disease.

11. Hyperthyroidism causes hyperreflexia and may occasionally also cause proximal myopathy.

12. Systolic flow murmurs may occur because of the high cardiac output.

13. It is polite to thank the patient. Always wash your hands to reduce the risk of cross-infection.

Examination Of A Goitre

		Not attempted	Attempted inadequate	Attempted adequate
1	Approaches the patient politely and introduces him/herself. Exposes the patient adequately after obtaining their permission.	0	1	2
2	Inspects the neck from the front and side, commenting on scars, prominent veins and whether any visible swelling is localised or generalised.	0	1	2
3	Asks the patient to swallow some water and comments on the movement of any lump in the neck.	0	1	2
4	Asks the patient to stick out their tongue and comments on the movement of any lump in the neck.	0	1	2
5	Asks the patient whether their neck is tender and then palpates the neck from behind. Asks the patient to swallow again whilst palpating. Comments on site, size, shape, consistency and mobility.	0	1	2
6	Palpates the cervical lymph nodes.	0	1	2
7	Palpates the carotid pulses.	0	1	2
8	Feels for deviation of the trachea.	0	1	2
9	Auscultates over each lobe for bruits.	0	1	2
10	Percusses over the sternal area for a retrosternal goitre.	0	1	2
11	Thanks patient and washes hands	0	1	2

1. It is important to introduce yourself (give your name and what you do) and explain that would like to examine their neck. Explain that you need to expose them fully in order to perform an adequate examination. Respect the modesty of patients. Explain what you are going to do as you proceed with the examination, *before* you do it!

2. A normal thyroid may be just visible in a thin person below the cricoid cartilage.
   A scar from a previous thyroidectomy may be visible.
   Prominent veins over the upper chest wall suggest retrosternal extension of the goitre causing thoracic inlet obstruction.

3. A goitre or a thyroglossal cyst will move on swallowing as they are attached to the larynx.

4. A thyroglossal cyst will move on poking out the tongue with the jaw stationary.

5. Site - a nodule may be obviously confined to one lobe.

   Size (WHO criteria):
   - 0 - no visible or palpable goitre.
   - 1a - goitre detectable only on palpation.
   - 1b - goitre palpable and visible only when neck is extended.
   - 2 - goitre visible with neck in normal position.
   - 3 - goitre visible from a distance.

Shape:
- Smooth or irregular?
- Diffuse or a single nodule?
- Can the lower margin be demarcated? (indicates absence of retrosternal extension).

Consistency:
- Soft (similar to fat) - normal.
- Firm (similar to muscle) - in a simple goitre.
- Hard (like a table top) - rubbery hard in Hashimoto's thyroiditis and stony hard in carcinoma, calcification in a cyst or fibrosis.

Mobility - the gland may be fixed by carcinoma.

6. Cervical lymph nodes may be involved in carcinoma of the thyroid.

7. Infiltration by a thyroid malignancy may occasionally render the carotid pulsation absent.

8. Deviation of the trachea may occur with a retrosternal goitre.

9. Bruits may be heard in goitres due to Graves' disease. Take care that it is not a carotid bruit being heard.

10. A change in percussion note over this area may mark out a retrosternal goitre.

11. It is polite to thank the patient. Always wash your hands to reduce the risk of cross-infection.

Examination Of The Diabetic Foot

		Not attempted	Attempted inadequate	Attempted adequate
1	Approaches the patient politely and introduces himself/herself. Exposes the patient adequately after obtaining their permission.	0	1	2
2	Inspects the legs for skin changes and muscle wasting.	0	1	2
3	Closely inspects the feet all over including between the toes. Comments on deformity, signs of peripheral vascular disease, ulceration, callus and signs of autonomic dysfunction.	0	1	2
4	Compares the temperature over the dorsum of each foot using the back of the hand.	0	1	2
5	Runs their hand up the sole of the foot to feel for any callus.	0	1	2
6	Palpates the foot pulses.	0	1	2
7	Tests the ankle jerk reflex.	0	1	2
8	Tests vibration sense in the peripheral joints.	0	1	2
9	Tests pinprick sensation in the feet.	0	1	2
10	Tests proprioception in the peripheral joints.	0	1	2
11	Asks the patient to walk if they are able.	0	1	2
12	Asks permission to assess the patient's footwear.	0	1	2
13	Thanks patient and washes hands	0	1	2

1. It is important to introduce yourself (give your name and what you do) and explain that would like to examine their legs and feet. Explain that you need to expose them fully (up to their thighs) in order to perform an adequate examination. Respect the modesty of patients. Explain what you are going to do as you proceed with the examination, *before* you do it!

2. Necrobiosis lipoidica diabeticorum is yellow / brown discolouration of the skin, usually over the shins, found in some people with DM.
   Wasting of quadriceps or tibialis anterior and the peroneal muscles due to neuropathy may be particularly noticeable.

3. Deformity may take the form of a claw foot with prominent metatarsal heads or the gross deformity of Charcot's joints (e.g. rocker bottom foot).
   Ischaemic discolouration (pale or dusky) is a sign of peripheral vascular disease. Ulcers may be arteriopathic, neuropathic or a combination of both. Arteriopathic ulcers typically occur on the tips of toes and the heels. Neuropathic ulcers form at sites of pressure eg. over the metatarsal heads.
   Callus is important to note because it acts as a foreign body and there is often underlying ulceration.
   Signs of autonomic dysfunction include dry skin, oedema and distended veins.

4. Warmth suggests active inflammation.
   Cold extremities occur in peripheral vascular disease.

5. This is a sensitive way of detecting callus, which may otherwise have been missed by inspection alone.

6. Absent peripheral pulses indicate peripheral vascular disease.
   Pulses in a neuropathic foot are often bounding.

7. Loss of this reflex occurs in diabetic peripheral neuropathy. If it is not present, go on to test the knee jerk reflex.

8. See the neurological examination sections for how to do this.
   If vibration sense is lost in the DIP joints, go on to test proximal joints.

9. Begin by demonstrating sharp and dull sensation to the patient in an area where they can feel it such as over the sternum.
   Then ask the patient to close their eyes and state whether they feel the sensation as sharp or dull when you prick their feet. Begin distally and work proximally to elicit the level of any peripheral neuropathy.

10. See the neurological examination sections for how to do this.
    Again, if an abnormality is detected, go on to test more proximal joints.

11. If the patient is able to walk, observing the gait can provide useful information.

12. This is an important part of the examination. Look to see whether there are irregularities or foreign bodies in the shoes and whether the style is suitable for a diabetic patient.

13. It is polite to thank the patient. Always wash your hands to reduce the risk of cross-infection.

The Genitourinary System

Urinary Tract History

		Not attempted	Attempted inadequate	Attempted adequate
1	Approaches patient politely and introduces him/herself.	0	1	2
2	Asks the patient's name, DOB and occupation.	0	1	2
3	Asks how many times a day the patient has to pass water on average.	0	1	2
4	Asks the patient how many times they have to get up at night to pass water.	0	1	2
5	Asks whether the patient feels they are passing more water than usual or whether they just have to go more often.	0	1	2
6	Asks whether the patient finds that when they get the urge to pass water, they have to rush to the toilet.	0	1	2
7	Asks whether the patient is ever incontinent of urine.	0	1	2
8	Asks if it is painful to pass water.	0	1	2
9	Asks whether the patient has ever noticed blood in their urine.	0	1	2
10	Asks whether the patient has difficulty in starting to pass water.	0	1	2
11	Asks whether the patient has noticed a decrease in the size of the stream.	0	1	2
12	Asks whether the patient ever gets terminal dribbling.	0	1	2
13	Asks about history of suprapubic or loin pain.	0	1	2
14	Asks whether the patient has had a fever or been shivering vigorously.	0	1	2
15	Asks about history of headache, vomiting, fits, drowsiness and peripheral oedema.	0	1	2
16	Asks whether the patient has noticed any weight loss.	0	1	2
17	Asks about relevant past or current conditions including UTIs, diabetes, gout, hypertension, ischaemic heart disease, and stroke.	0	1	2
18	Asks about family history of diabetes, hypertension and polycystic kidney disease.	0	1	2
19	Asks about smoking and alcohol consumption.	0	1	2
20	Asks about home circumstances.	0	1	2
21	Asks about past and current medications and any allergies to medication.	0	1	2

1. It is polite to introduce yourself and explain your task.

2. Name: to establish rapport and identify the patient.
   Age/DOB: certain diseases affect certain age groups, e.g. urothelial tumours are rare below the age of 40. The date of birth should be recorded to identify the patient.
   Occupation: workers in the rubber and dye industries are at increased risk of bladder cancer.

3. The need to urinate more often than normal is known as frequency. It can be due to the bladder being irritable (infection, inflammation, chemical irritation), less compliant (fibrosis, tumour infiltration) or to bladder outflow obstruction.

4. Most people do not need to get up during the night to pass urine. If someone is getting up more than once on regular occasions a cause should be looked for.

5. This distinguishes between polyuria and frequency.
   Polyuria can be due to ingestion of large volumes of fluid (especially alcohol), inability to concentrate the urine (chronic renal failure, hypercalcaemia or diabetes insipidus), diabetes mellitus or diuretics.

6. Urgency is a sign of an unstable bladder. It can occur in urinary tract infection, bladder cancer or bladder irritability.

7. Urinary incontinence is common in women as they get older. By the age of 60, 15-20% of women are incontinent at least once a week.
   Urge incontinence is characterised by urgency and frequency and is due to detrusor instability. It can be motor (where the urge to urinate before the bladder is full is due to an abnormality of the motor system such as MS) or sensory (where irritation is making the bladder unstable).
   Stress incontinence is where leakage occurs in response to increased abdominal pressure (coughing, laughing or sneezing) without contraction of detrusor. Damage to the bladder neck supports during childbirth and stretching of the ligaments during pregnancy predispose to stress incontinence.
   Urge and stress incontinence may occur together and the two cannot be easily distinguished clinically.

8. The most common cause of a stinging or burning sensation on passing urine is cystitis. However, dysuria can also be caused by stones and bladder cancer.

9. See specific history for haematuria.

10. - 12. Hesitancy, poor stream and terminal dribbling are classed as voiding symptoms and are signs of bladder outflow obstruction. This is common in men and usually due to an enlarged prostate. Associated symptoms include frequency and nocturia.
   In women, obstruction may be due to a pelvic cancer.
   Other substances, such as a calculus, clot or tumour can also cause obstruction.

13. Pyelonephritis causes pain and tenderness in the renal angles, usually in association with urinary symptoms and systemic illness.
   Renal stones can also cause loin pain.
   Ureteric stones cause colicky pain radiating from loin to groin. This is an intense pain associated with nausea, vomiting and sweating.
   Bladder stones cause dull suprapubic discomfort associated with dysuria and frequency.

14. Pyrexia and rigors occur in acute pyelonephritis. An infected, obstructed kidney can progress to gram negative septicaemia and is an emergency.

15. These are symptoms of uraemia.

16. Significant weight loss may be a sign of malignancy.

17. UTIs in childhood can scar the kidneys or may indicate that there is an underlying abnormality. In adult males UTIs are rare and need investigating. In females they are fairly common but it is important to exclude an underlying cause if they occur frequently.
Gout can be precipitated by renal impairment.
Diabetes has renal complications.
Hypertension can damage the kidneys and in some cases, renal disease may be the underlying cause.
A history of cardiovascular or cerebrovascular disease implies that renovascular disease ought to be considered.

18. Polycystic kidney disease is an autosomal dominant condition.
Diabetes and hypertension often occur in members of the same family although the pattern of inheritance is not straightforward.

19. Smoking is a major risk factor for urothelial tumours.
Alcohol can cause polyuria.

20. This can provide insight as to how the patient will cope with having a chronic illness and what form of support they have available.

21. Analgesic abuse can cause renal failure.
Certain drugs can worsen renal function when it is already abnormal including tetracycline and aminoglycoside antibiotics and NSAIDs.
Rifampicin can cause red discolouration of the urine.
Tricyclic antidepressants and lithium can cause incontinence.

Presenting Complaint - Haematuria

		Not attempted	Attempted inadequate	Attempted adequate
1	Asks the patient when they first noticed blood in their urine.	0	1	2
2	Asks if it was an isolated occasion or whether it is a regular occurrence.	0	1	2
3	Asks whether they passed frank blood or if it was just a small amount colouring the urine.	0	1	2
4	Asks the patient whether the haematuria is associated with pain and if so, asks relevant details about the pain.	0	1	2
5	Asks the patient whether the blood is at the start, the end or all the way through the stream.	0	1	2
6	Asks about symptoms of urgency and frequency.	0	1	2
7	Asks about symptoms of hesitancy, poor stream and terminal dribbling.	0	1	2
8	Asks whether the patient has noticed any weight loss.	0	1	2
9	Asks about past history of prostatic disease, stones, urinary tract infections, TB, and bleeding disorders.	0	1	2
10	Asks about family history of renal tract abnormalities.	0	1	2
11	Asks specifically about exposure to aromatic hydrocarbons (rubber and dye industry).	0	1	2
12	Asks whether the patient smokes.	0	1	2
13	Asks whether the patient takes any medications, in particular rifampicin or anticoagulants.	0	1	2

1. It is important to find out about the time course of the haematuria.

2. This allows assessment of the chronicity and severity of the haematuria.

3. This helps gauge the amount of blood that is being lost.

4. Painless haematuria is the commonest presenting complaint of bladder malignancy. Associated loin pain or ureteric colic suggests that a stone or clot (often associated with a tumour) is the cause.
   Suprapubic pain with haematuria points to a bladder stone as the cause.

6. Blood at the end of micturition suggests bleeding from the prostate or bladder base. Bleeding throughout the stream suggests that the blood comes from the bladder or above.
   Bleeding at the start of the stream but with the urine then running clear suggests a urethral lesion.

7. These symptoms are common in urinary tract infection, which can cause haematuria.

8. These are symptoms of obstruction, which is commonly due to prostatic enlargement (benign prostatic hypertrophy or prostatic carcinoma). The dilated veins around the prostate can rupture leading to haematuria.

9. Significant recent weight loss in the context of haematuria is a sinister sign.

10. Stones and urinary tract infections have a tendency to recur.
    The urinary tract can be affected by TB following haematogenous spread from other sites.
    Schistosomiasis infection leads to chronic bladder inflammation and is a risk factor for squamous cell carcinoma.
    Bleeding disorders can cause haematuria.

11. Haematuria can be a feature of polycystic kidney disease if there is haemorrhage into a cyst.

12. This is a risk factor for renal and bladder cancer.

13. Smoking is a major risk factor for urothelial tumours.

14. Overdose of anticoagulants can lead to bleeding.
    Rifamipicin can cause red discoloration of the urine.

Sexual Medical History

		Not attempted	Attempted inadequate	Attempted adequate
1	Approaches the patient politely and introduces him/herself.	0	1	2
2	Asks the patient's name, DOB and occupation.	0	1	2
3	Asks the reason for attendance.	0	1	2
4	Asks whether the patient has noticed any urethral discharge.	0	1	2
5	Asks whether they have noticed any ulcers and if so whether they are painful.	0	1	2
6	Asks whether they have any rash or itching.	0	1	2
7	Asks whether passing water is painful.	0	1	2
8	Asks whether sexual intercourse is painful.	0	1	2
9	Asks about the patient's sexual orientation and gets an accurate description of sexual practices.	0	1	2
10	Asks when the patient last had sex and whether it was with a regular partner.	0	1	2
11	Asks whether their partner has any symptoms.	0	1	2
12	Asks whether the patient uses contraception and if so, what form.	0	1	2
13	Asks the date of the patient's last menstrual period.	0	1	2
14	Asks whether the patient is up to date on her smear tests and whether she has ever had any abnormal results.	0	1	2
15	Asks if the patient has ever injected drugs and if so, whether they shared needles.	0	1	2
16	Asks if the patient has ever had sex with someone from abroad.	0	1	2
17	Asks if the patient has ever had sex with a prostitute.	0	1	2
18	Asks if they have ever had a blood transfusion.	0	1	2
19	Asks about relevant past or current conditions including previous sexually transmitted infections, UTIs, diabetes or cold sores.	0	1	2
20	Asks about smoking and alcohol consumption.	0	1	2
21	Asks about home circumstances.	0	1	2
22	Asks about past and current medications and any allergies to medication.	0	1	2

1. It is polite to introduce yourself and explain your task. Obtaining a sexual history requires discretion and tact.

2. Name: to establish rapport and identify the patient. In this situation though, the patient may not wish to give their name.

   Age/DOB: the date of birth should be recorded to identify the patient. If the patient is female and under 16 years old, there may be issues of child protection to consider if she is sexually active.

   Occupation: this provides information about the patient's background and can have significant effects on the management of their condition.

3. It is important to establish whether the patient is attending because of his or her own symptoms, because a partner has had symptoms or because their name was given in the contact-tracing scheme.

4. In men, urethral discharge is commonly caused by gonorrhoea, chlamydia, trichomonas or candida. However, there are other causes and in 25% of cases no cause is identified and it is known as non-specific urethritis.
   See specific history for vaginal discharge.

5. The commonest cause of multiple painful genital ulcers is herpes simplex infection. Syphilis causes a solitary painless ulcer. (Syphilis in babies causes 'snuffles') Carcinoma can also cause painless ulceration.

6. Candida albicans and trichomonas vaginalis infections can lead to vulvovaginitis. Warts can sometimes lead to itching and burning.

7. Dysuria is a symptom of urinary tract infection but also occurs in urethritis due to gonorrhoea infection.

8. Dyspareunia can be caused by infection, endometriosis, vaginal dryness (at the menopause) or psychological factors.

9. The differential diagnosis varies according to whether the patient is practising anal or oral sex and whether they are insertive, receptive or both.

10. This is important both for finding out what level of risk the patient is at and for contact tracing.

11. This can provide clues as to the organisms that may have been passed on to this patient and is also important because their partner could be unaware that they are infective.

12. The importance of good contraception should be stressed and advice can be given at this stage. It is important to emphasise the need for condoms for protection against sexually transmitted infections.

13. If there is any possibility of pregnancy, management of any infections may alter and options will need to be discussed with the patient.

14. If the patient is not up to date on her smear tests she should be advised to see her GP once any infection has been treated.

15-18. These are risk factors for HIV and hepatitis B infection. Put the patient at ease by explaining that these questions are asked routinely.

19. Diabetes predisposes to infection, especially if poorly controlled.
   Urinary tract infections have a tendency to recur in some women and can be precipitated by sexual intercourse.
   Cold sores are usually caused by herpes simplex type 1, whereas genital herpes is usually herpes simplex type 2. However, these divisions are not rigid and herpes simplex type 1 can sometimes also cause genital lesions.

20. Smoking is a risk factor for cervical carcinoma.

21. Home circumstances can affect treatment compliance.

22. Find out which medications the patient has tried in the past and whether any caused allergic reactions.

Presenting Complaint - Vaginal Discharge

		Not attempted	Attempted inadequate	Attempted adequate
1	Asks whether the patient has noticed an increase in the amount of vaginal discharge.	0	1	2
2	Asks whether the discharge has an odour.	0	1	2
3	Asks what colour the discharge is and whether there is any blood in it.	0	1	2
4	Asks whether there is an associated itch.	0	1	2
5	Asks whether they have any pain on passing water.	0	1	2
6	Asks whether they have any abdominal or pelvic pain.	0	1	2
7	Asks whether sexual intercourse is painful.	0	1	2
8	Asks whether the patient has felt unwell, for example with a fever and malaise.	0	1	2
9	Asks whether the patient has recently changed sexual partner and whether her partner has any symptoms.	0	1	2
10	Asks what form of contraception the patient uses.	0	1	2
11	Asks the date of the patient's last menstrual period.	0	1	2
12	Asks whether the patient is up to date on her smear tests and whether she has ever had any abnormal results.	0	1	2
13	Asks whether they have ever had any sexually transmitted infections in the past.	0	1	2
14	Asks whether the patient is on antibiotics for any reason.	0	1	2

1. Physiological causes of increased discharge include puberty, pregnancy, ovulation, and the combined oral contraceptive pill.
   Pathological causes include infection, a foreign body, an ectropion, a polyp or malignancy.

2. Bacterial vaginosis and trichomonas are associated with a fishy smelling discharge.

3. Candida infection causes a thick white discharge.
   Bacterial vaginosis causes a thin grey discharge.
   Trichomonas vaginalis causes a greenish frothy discharge.
   Gonorrhoea causes a white / yellow discharge.
   Chlamydia infection isn't usually associated with a discharge but if it ascends to cause pelvic inflammatory disease, a watery or muco-purulent discharge can occur.
   A bloody discharge can be a feature of an ectropion or an endocervical polyp.

4. Candida and trichomonas infection can both cause itch.

5. Gonorrhoea can cause urethritis, which can lead to dysuria.
   Alternatively, the patient may have an associated urinary tract infection causing this symptom.

6. Pelvic inflammatory disease (most commonly due to chlamydia infection) causes low abdominal pain in association with discharge.

7. Dyspareunia can be associated with vulvo-vaginitis of any cause but is also a common feature of pelvic inflammatory disease.

8. Patients with pelvic inflammatory disease will be systemically unwell.

9. This suggests that a sexually transmitted infection might be the cause e.g. trichomonas, gonorrhoea or chlamydia.

10. This is a good opportunity to offer contraceptive advice if needed.

11. It is important to establish whether the patient might be pregnant.

12. Cervical cancer is a very rare cause of vaginal discharge but again, this is a good opportunity to encourage the patient to attend for regular smear tests.

13. A past history of chlamydia suggests that pelvic inflammatory disease should be considered.
    Recurrent candida infection should prompt consideration as to whether there is an underlying cause e.g. resistant organisms or diabetes.

14. Broad-spectrum antibiotics predispose to candida infection.

COMMUNICATION

Informed Consent

		Not done	Adequate	Good
1	Introduces self and role and identifies patient by name and date of birth	0	1	2
2	Explains reason for the interview.	0	1	2
3	Assesses the patient's starting point	0	1	2
4	Explores options of treatment with patient and discusses pros and cons of each option.	0	1	2
5	Facilitates patient to make their own choice	0	1	2
6	Demonstrates appropriate non-verbal behaviour	0	1	2
7	"Chunks and checks" using patient response to guide following steps	0	1	2
8	Discovers what other information would help the patient	0	1	2
9	Gives explanation in an organised manner	0	1	2
10	Checks patient's understanding	0	1	2
11	Uses clear language	0	1	2
12	Encourages patient to contribute	0	1	2
13	Notices and responds to non verbal cues	0	1	2
14	Demonstrates professionalism and compassion	0	1	2
		0	1	2

1. It is both polite, rapport building and necessary to greet a patient and confirm their identity. It is best to do this with both their name and, if available their date of birth.
2. It is important the patient knows both who you are and your role. They must understand whether you are a doctor or a student, and whether you are here only to gain consent or to play a part in the procedure as well. Explain the reason for the interview, in that you are going to discuss the available treatments for their condition.
3. Many patients will have some idea of what the proposed or potential treatment options are. Explore what they already know and ask them if they wish to explore the options. The candidate must gauge what the patient already understands about the procedure and the patient's preference for the amount of further information to be given.

4. The patient has the right to have the options fully explored, including any dilemmas that may present themselves, whilst the doctor has to signpost position of equipoise (the possibility that there are other options out there). It is important to discuss the advantages and disadvantages of each option of treatment and help the patient in making their own decision which they are happy with. There is a need to rapidly establish the level of involvement the patient wishes to have in the decision making process and if appropriate should be encouraged to make all their own choices and decisions.

5. You should show a clear interest and concern for the patient as a person through empathic statements, "I know this can seem a bit daunting/anxiety provoking etc" and by not in anyway being overtly offensive or judgemental. Often patients ask 'what do you think doctor': The response to this has to be your own opinion followed by the reasons for that opinion.

6. Non verbal behaviour includes good eye contact, posture and position, movements, mirroring and use of voice in both tone and volume.

7. 'Chunks and checks' implies repeatedly pausing, whilst gauging the patients response before moving on and allowing the responses that are forthcoming to guide the next steps in the explanation.

8. One should make a careful effort to seek and address and specific needs the patient might have.

9. The explanation should contain overt use of both summarising and signposting

10. You can simply ask the patient to restate any information given so far.

11. Clear language should be used throughout, with minimal use of jargon.

12. You should actively encourage the patient to contribute and responds well to any concerns they might have, exploring them as needed.

13. The candidate should be sensitive to the patient's non-verbal or verbal cues; hand wringing, appearing nervous, and phrases such as "so what are the risks again?"

14. It is important that throughout the patient must not feel coerced or pressured.

Explaining a Procedure

		Not done	Adequate	Good
1	Introduces self and your role, as well as the purpose of the consultation. Identifies patient by name and date of birth.			
2	Explores what the patient knows already			
3	Clarifies the name and basic nature of the procedure.			
4	Explains any basic anatomy or physiology that may need clarifying			
5	Clarifies the indications for the procedure			
6	Explores any contraindications to the procedure			
7	Discusses the risks, benefits and any possible alternatives. Quantifies risk as much as possible.			
8	Discusses the equipment involved in the procedure			
9	Explains the basic way in which the procedure will progress			
10	Explains post-procedure care, including follow-up			
11	Responds empathically to any anxieties, worries or concerns exhibited by the patient			
12	Checks understanding			
13	Allows for pauses and invites questions from the patient at appropriate intervals			
14	Has an organised approach to the consultation			

Breaking Bad News

		Not done	Adequate	Good
1	Confirms correct environment			
2	Greets patient and confirms patient's name and date of birth and address			
3	Introduces self and role			
4	Explains nature of interview			
5	Assesses the patient's starting point and what they know already			
6	Gives clear signposting that serious and important information is to follow			
7	"Chunks and checks" using patient response to guide following steps			
8	Discovers what other information would help patient			
9	Gives explanation in organised manner			
10	Uses clear language			
11	Picks up and responds to non-verbal cues			
12	Allows patient time to react.			
13	Encourages patient to contribute			
14	Acknowledges patients concerns and feelings			
15	Uses empathy to communicate appreciation of the patients feelings or predicament			
16	Demonstrates appropriate non-verbal behaviour			
17	Provides support			
18	Makes appropriate arrangement for follow up contact.			

1. Choose a time that is not busy, a quiet room away from the ward if possible. Ask if the patient wants anyone with them.
2. It is both polite, rapport building and necessary to greet a patient and confirm their identity. It is best to do this with both their name and, if available their date of birth and address. Giving bad news to the wrong patient is a terrible mistake to make!
3. It is important to make it clear who you are and what your role is within the team responsible for their care.
4. It is vital that the patient knows the reason for you coming to talk to the patient, "I have come to talk about the results of the tests you had" but also vital in these situations to give the appropriate gravity to explanation.
5. You need to explore what the patient knows and understands already, "What have you already been told about might be going on?"
6. Honest disclosure of information allows patients to make informed decisions that are consistent with their goals, values and expectations. When physicians withhold bad news, they diminish patient autonomy.

7. 'Chunks and checks' implies repeatedly pausing, whilst gauging the patients response before moving on and allowing the responses that are forthcoming to guide the next steps in the explanation.

8. You must attempt to address the patients individual information needs, "Are you the sort of person who likes to know all the details of your condition?" or "Would you like me to discuss the results of the CT scan with you?" You simply need to attempt to address these concerns, but should not be expected to necessarily know the answer.

9. The explanation should contain overt use of both summarising and signposting. Avoid euphemisms, bluntness but equally avoid "dancing around the topic".

10. Clear language should be used throughout, with minimal use of jargon or confusing language.

11. The candidate should be sensitive to the patient's non-verbal cues, especially crying, looking for help etc.

12. Possibly the most important aspect of the consultation, the candidate should allow for long silences if need be, otherwise known as "shut down" moments. It is important to tune into patient readiness to hear more, and knowing when to stop.

13. You should ask about their concerns and feeling in an empathic manner while watching for their nonverbal reactions. You can name the feelings and respond in a respectful manner, "I know this is upsetting, but it would be for anyone". Or 'it may seem easy for me to say …'

14. These concerns and feels should be acknowledged even if their values are different from your own. You should accept their legitimacy in their own right.

15. Observe for and allow emotional reactions, with kleenex handy and appropriate use of touch. Supportive phrases can also be helpful at this stage, "I'll do everything I can to help you through this."

16. Non-verbal behaviour includes good eye contact, posture and position, movements, mirroring and use of voice in both tone and volume as well as appropriate use of touch.

17. At this juncture it is ideal to express concern, understanding and a willingness to help.

18. Summarize discussion with a clear follow-up plan re: referral, tests, next contact (in <48 hrs). You can also offer to provide written summary or brochures. Invite a support person for next visit if not present.

Post Mortem Consent

		Not done	Adequate	Good
1	Introduces self and confirms the identity of both the relative and their relationship to the patient			
2	Sensitively and empathically explores how the relative is feeling. Appreciates this is a difficult time for them			
3	Confirms next of kin and clarifies whether other members of the family would wish to be present			
4	Explores what the relative knows about the purpose of your consultation			
5	Gives reasons for performing a post mortem			
6	Makes absolutely clear that they can refuse consent			
7	Explores relative's knowledge of PMs			
8	Offers and give any further information the relative requires.			
9	Clarifies any preference towards burial or cremation and whether the deceased was of a particular faith			
10	Gives explanation in organised manner			
11	Uses clear language			
12	Uses empathy to communicate appreciation of the patients feelings or predicament			
13	Provides support			
14	Confirms consent.			

1. It is both polite, rapport building and necessary to greet a relative and confirm their identity and their relationship to the deceased.
2. This is something that needs to be done very sensitively. Do not simply launch into a potentially highly emotional and devastating discussion. An excellent technique is to phrase your opening statements along the lines of, "I am sorry to hear about the loss of your relative. How are you feeling now? I can see you are upset/worn out/etc. It is very kind of you to speak to me at this difficult time".
3. It is acceptable to simply ask if the relative is the next of kin and if not to ask whether there are any close family members about.
4. Clarify your role in the team. It will be highly likely that you will have been asked by a senior to speak the relative about a post mortem examination. Make sure they know that this is the purpose of the consultation. The candidate should allow for long silences if need be, otherwise known as "shut down" moments. It is important to tune into relative's readiness to hear more, and knowing when to stop.
5. Begin by being general in your explanation, "Although we are relatively sure of the cause of death, there are things which are not very clear and the only way to answer these questions is to perform a hospital post mortem."
   Be aware a *Coroner's* PM is ordered in the case of a sudden or unexpected death where the cause is not 100% clear and a death certificate cannot be issued, or if the cause is other than a natural disease
   Deaths must be referred to the coroner if
   - The cause is unknown

- The practitioner has not attended the deceased during their last illness
- The practitioner neither attended the deceased during the last 14 days before death nor saw the body after death.
- Negligence could be alleged in the patients death

In a hospital PM, there is no delay in the issuing of a death certificate and it is for purely academic purposes.

6. Make it clear that a HOSPITAL post mortem is completely for academic interest and that the family can refuse consent. However, make it clear that post mortems help advance medical understanding of certain conditions and help pick up ways in which these conditions might me better treated.
7. Clarify if the relative would like to know more and off. You must attempt to address the patients individual information needs. Use the 'Chunks and checks' method, by repeatedly pausing, whilst gauging the patients response before moving on and allowing the responses that are forthcoming to guide the next steps in the explanation
8. If so you should inform them that;
    a. It is a careful and respectful internal examination of the body
    b. It is carried out as soon as possible after consent is given
    c. It is carried out by a pathologist, assisted by a qualified technician
    d. Photos and x-rays may be taken.
    e. An incision is made from collarbone to the 'tummy' and at the back of the head. Reassure that these will not be visible once the body has been dressed. The organs will b removed and return to the body immediately after the examination. Be very careful in choosing to deliver these gory details!
    f. Clarify that some tissue may be retained for analysis but that they will be informed and asked for permission if this is the case.
    g. The body can be cremated or buried after PM.
    h. It can take up to 3 hours.
9. It is important to find out if the deceased had specifically expressed any preferences and was known to have a specific faith which requires any special considerations to be made.
10. The explanation should contain overt use of both summarising and signposting. Avoid euphemisms, bluntness but equally avoid "dancing around the topic".
11. Clear language should be used throughout, with minimal use of jargon or confusing language
12. Invite questions and elucidate any new worries or concerns that may have arisen.
13. You should ask about their concerns and feeling in an empathic manner while watching for their nonverbal reactions. You can name the feelings and respond in a respectful manner
14. Use a phrase such as "Do I have your approval for this post mortem to be carried out on your mother in the fashion I have described?" Offer to keep them updated as more information becomes available.

Drug Adherence

		Not done	Adequate	Good
1	Introduces self and explains role	0	1	2
2	Clarifies the reason for the consultation	0	1	2
3	Establishes the patients understanding of the proposed treatment	0	1	2
4	Explores the treatment fully, including a) Reason for being on the medication b) How long the patient has been on it and how long they are likely to be on it c) The benefits of being on the medication d) The possible side effects of the treatment e) What to do in case of side effects f) Why it is important to take this medication as directed g) Is there any monitoring involved (i.e. blood levels, peak flows etc) h) Any possible drug interactions i) If an acute medication (e.g. insulin, salbutamol) the need to have it nearby at all times j) Any legal ramifications of the treatment (e.g. antiepileptics)	0	1	2
5	Does the above in a simple manner, avoiding jargon	0	1	2
6	Responds empathically to any anxieties, worries or concerns exhibited by the patient	0	1	2
7	Checks understanding	0	1	2
8	Allows for pauses and invites questions from the patient at appropriate intervals	0	1	2
9	Has an organised approach to the consultation	0	1	2

1. It is polite to introduce yourself and explain your role.
2. This allows you to prepare the patient for the interview and develop rapport
3. This can be done in an open fashion, such as "So tell me about the medications you are on", or if you feel that time is an issue, in a more closed fashion, "Tell me what you know about your asthma medication"
4.
    a. You must discern the medical reason for their being on the treatment in a concise manner, "So why were you started on warfarin"
    b. Some drugs are only a short term consideration, such as prednisolone in an asthma exacerbation, whereas a patient on warfarin or insulin may have been on it for years and may have to stay on it for years to come.
    c. Many patients struggle to "see" the benefits of the medication they are on. You have to clarify this, as adherence will increase once a patient understands why they are actually taking an inhaler, pill or injection.

d. These are frequently a reason for poor compliance but you must explore whether the patient understands that is a side effect. How severe is it? Will it fade over time? Are there ways around it?

e. For example bleeding heavily in a warfarinised patient versus a patient suffering shaking after taking their inhaler. You must clarify he difference between a mild side effect and one that you may be concerned about.

f. It is your responsibility to educate the patient as to why the regime prescribed is important to adhere to. There are frequently reasons for this, whether it be taking a statin at night or taking a bisphosphonate at the same time each week.

g. Do they need to attend clinics or go to their GP for monitoring? Many medications require some form of monitoring either in the form of blood tests, (INR for anticoagulation, Lithium levels etc) or perhaps other means, (BP in antihypertensives, PEFR with a new inhaler)

h. Does their medication interact with other drugs, foods or alcohol?

i. Many adherence issues are based around a patient not appreciating that they must have their inhaler/epi-pen, insulin etc on their person or near them at all times. This can sometime be quite an upheaval for the patient and difficult for them to do.

j. Do they need to tell any organisations that they are now on this medication? This can include the DVLA, their work or employer etc.

5. This consultation is an exercise in education and thus must be done in a fashion that the patient can understand

6. Issues of adherence can sometimes be very upsetting for a patient. A young patient may hate the idea of having to inject himself with insulin every day. You must respond appropriately.

7. Stop and ask them if all has been made clear. You can ask them to repeat information back to you and even off to write it down for them.

8. You must give the patient time to think and consider whether they feel they need any further clarification of a point

9. Working in a systematic manner will make this process easier for you and the patient

Cardio-Pulmonary Resuscitation

Adult Cardio-Pulmonary Resuscitation (CPR)

		Not attempted	Attempted inadequate	Attempted adequate
1	Ensures a safe approach	0	1	2
2	Shouts for help/pulls emergency buzzer	0	1	2
3	Assesses for responsiveness	0	1	2
4	Opens airway & look for visible obstruction	0	1	2
5	Checks for breathing & pulse for 10 seconds	0	1	2
6	Ensures 2222 is called	0	1	2
7	Sends staff for emergency equipment	0	1	2
8	Commences 30 chest compressions:			
	Correct depth 4-5cm	0	1	2
	Correct rate 100/min	0	1	2
	Correct position	0	1	2
9	Administers 2 effective ventilations (**must** use airway adjunct)	0	1	2
10	Ensures oxygen 15 litres used with airway adjunct	0	1	2
11	Continues at 30:2 ratio demonstrating effective CPR	0	1	2
The cardiac monitor arrives:				
12	**What is the rhythm ?** Ventricular Fibrillation	0	0	1
13	**What treatment is now required?** 1.Defibrillation 1 shock, 150-360J biphasic or 360J monophasic 2. Immediately resume 2 min CPR 30:2	0	0	1
14	Wash hands when concluded			

1. A safe approach is where the victim, bystanders and the person doing the CPR is safe and away from danger (e.g., away from traffic etc) and in hospital, there is enough room around the bed/couch to perform CPR safely.

2.It is important to shout for help, especially experienced help. In a ward situation, it is important to call any available medical or nursing staff.

3. Responsiveness is assessed by gently shaking the victim and asking 'are you all right'.

4. An obvious cause for airway obstruction (e.g., a food bolus) must be sought before commencing CPR.

5. Loss of pulse and respiratory effort indicate cardiopulmonary arrest. If a pulse is present, emphasis can be placed on respiratory support.

6. 2222 is the usual call number for in-hospital arrests and ensures that the a cardiac arrest call out is immediately sent to the resuscitation team.

7. An emergency trolley with airway, intubation equipment and emergency drugs is usually available in every clinical area.

8. 30 chest compressions followed by 2 effective ventilations (by bag and mask or mouth-to-mouth) is the recommended ratio. Place the heel of one hand on the centre of the chest, place the other hand on top and interlock the fingers of both hands. Keep your arms straight and your fingers off the chest and use the weight of your body to apply compressions to a depth of 5cm. Then release the pressure and repeat at a rate of 100/min.

9. An airway adjunct is an aid to keeping the airway open (e.g., Guadal airway)

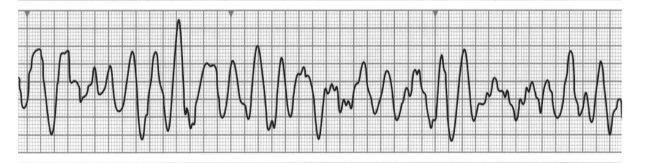

PAEDIATRIC BASIC LIFE SUPPORT
(For healthcare professionals with a duty to respond)

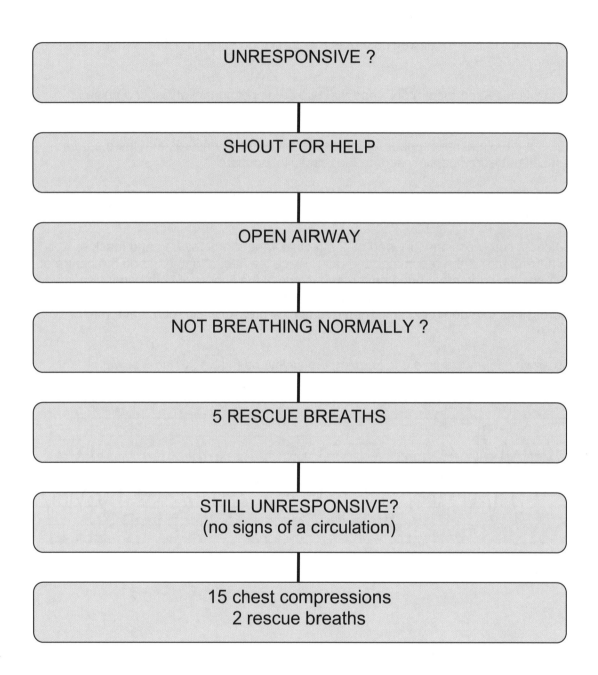

UNRESPONSIVE ?

SHOUT FOR HELP

OPEN AIRWAY

NOT BREATHING NORMALLY ?

5 RESCUE BREATHS

STILL UNRESPONSIVE?
(no signs of a circulation)

15 chest compressions
2 rescue breaths

After 1 minute call resuscitation team then continue CPR

(http://www.resus.org.uk/pages/pblsalgo.pdf)

PROCEDURES

Handwashing and Scrubbing Up

		Not performed	Performed inadequately	Performed adequately
1	If handwashing is preceding scrubbing up, ensure correct theatre clothing is worn, a freshly donned face mask, all hair covered under cap and no jewellery except plain wedding rings. Ensure sterile theatre wear is set up for use after the scrub	0	1	2
2	Wet hands and dispense scrub solution into the palm of the hand using elbows to work dispenser. Wash hands and forearms thoroughly.	0	1	2
3	Palm to palm	0	1	2
4	Right palm over back of left hand. Change hands and repeat	0	1	2
5	Interlace fingers of right hand over left. Change hands and repeat.	0	1	2
6	Rotational rubbing of right hand in left palm. Change hands and repeat.	0	1	2
7	Rotational rubbing of right thumb clasped in left palm. Change hands and repeat	0	1	2
8	Grasp left wrist with right hand and work cleanser into skin. Change hands and repeat	0	1	2
9	Rub hands and wrists for 30 seconds, then rinse and dry thoroughly.	0	1	2
10	Take (impregnated) nail brush and scrub nails thoroughly. Brushing other areas of the hands and is detrimental to the skin surface, causing abrasions. The brush should be used for the first session only.	0	1	2
11	After 2 minutes, rinse, keeping hands higher than elbows	0	1	2
12	Re-apply scrub solution and continue to wash for a further 3 minutes from fingers to forearms	0	1	2
13	Turn off taps using elbow controls and allow arms to drip into sink before turning to the opened gown pack.	0	1	2
14	Subsequent scrub involves a 3 minute wash from fingers to mid forearm	0	1	2
15	The skin should be blotted dry. Adhering to the principle that it is important to work from fingertips to elbows	0	1	2
16	Open the inner gown wrap, take folded towel, open like a book. Place on palm of hand and dry the fingers, palm and back of opposite hand thoroughly	0	1	2

17	Protecting the other hand with the towel, grasp the wrist and corkscrew spiral down the arm to dry it, ending at the elbow	0	1	2
18	Replace the towel and repeat for the other hand and arm without contaminating hands	0	1	2
19	Pick up the gown and let the bottom unfold. Keep your hands on the inside and ensure the ties do not flap from the unsterile to the sterile side	0	1	2
20	Open the gown and put your hands inside the sleeves simultaneously. Keep your hands inside the sleeves	0	1	2
21	The scrub nurse should ease the gown on you from behind, and fasten the poppers or tie the strings	0	1	2
22	Once gowned, the candidate will secure the side fastening on wrap around gowns by: - Removing the left hand cord. - Handing the card to scrub nurse. - Rotating anti clockwise and fastening at front	0	1	2
23	Take the gloves from the sterile packet, opened by the scrub nurse , by opening out the packet and picking up one glove by its cuff	0	1	2
24	Lay the glove on the palm of the hand with the fingers pointing up the arm, with the thumb of the glove to your thumb inside the sleeve	0	1	2
25	Hold the cuff of the glove thumb to thumb. With the other hand, pull the cuff over the sleeve and slide your fingers through and into the glove. Do this away from you at arms length and not up near your mask	0	1	2
26	If gloves require changing intra-operatively because of puncture, the completion of a dirty procedure or inadvertent contamination, this should be done using a closed gloving technique (or plunge gloving technique)	0	1	2

1.   The scrub practitioner should ensure:-

    a. All hair is covered under the theatre hat or hood.
    b. Theatre clothing (scrubbed suits) is secured. No other clothing i.e. gowns, should be worn.
    c. A freshly donned face mask is correctly positioned over the nose and mouth and fitted comfortably. For all intermediate and major surgery theatre personnel are advised to wear masks for *their own protection*
    d. Hands and nails are clean, nails are short and free from all nail varnish.
    e. The wearing of jewellery is actively discouraged other than a wedding band.

f. Spectacles and microscopic glasses are positioned and secured prior to surgery.

g. The skin is intact on hands and arms and are free from abrasions. Very small cuts or blemishes must be covered with a sterile plaster after scrubbing up.

h. Protective clothing - lead or plastic aprons are donned and comfortable, prior to scrubbing up.

2-9.

A variety of skin disinfecting solutions will be provided, eg. Betadine, Hibiscrub etc. It is useful to follow a pattern to ensure that all areas of hands and forearms are cleansed thoroughly.

10-14.

The first scrub **must** take 5 minutes with subsequent scrubs taking 3 minutes.

The scrub practitioner should be aware that the purpose of the scrub procedure is to attack the transient and resident micro-organisms on the hands and forearms

In order to minimise contamination during the scrubbing procedure staff should ensure at all times:-

i. The water should be at an even temperature and steady flow.

ii. The hands are above the level of the elbows.

iii. Care is taken not to splash theatre clothing.

v. Rinsing is performed from fingertips to elbows, using the water flow and not hands. Vigorous shaking to dispel water from hands and arms is unacceptable.

Brushing other areas of the hands and arms has shown to be detrimental to the skin surface causing abrasions.

15-18.

The skin should be blotted dry with sterile disposable paper towels. Rubbing the skin in order to dry it, will disturb skin cells.

19-26

It is essential that staff discard any gown that is either too small or too big for their use. Both are unsafe.

The scrub practitioner must ensure that he/she touches the INSIDE of the gown only and both arms are inserted into the sleeves of the gown simultaneously.

Arterial Blood Gas

		Not Attempted	Attempted inadequate	Attempted adequate
1.	Introduces him/herself to patient, gains consent	0	1	2
2.	Assembles and prepares appropriate equipment	0	1	2
3.	Identifies patient verbally and using I.D bracelet	0	1	2
4.	Washes hands and wears gloves	0	1	2
5.	Identifies radial artery site	0	1	2
6.	Performs Allens test	0	1	2
7.	Palpates artery for maximum pulsation	0	1	2
8.	Cleans site with an alcohol swab and allows for 30 seconds or until dry	0	1	2
9.	Fully extend the patients wrist	0	1	2
10.	Holds syringe at 45° angle (must point in opposite direction of arterial flow)	0	1	2
11.	Performs arterial blood sampling using correct technique	0	1	2
12.	Ensures pressure is maintained until patient stops bleeding	0	1	2
13.	Remove needle in an appropriate manner discarding into sharps bin	0	1	2
14.	Expels air and applies cap	0	1	2
15.	Mixes sample	0	1	2
16.	Mentions syringe labelling and that they would send for immediate analysis	0	1	2
17.	Disposes of equipment safely	0	1	2
18.	Does all the above in a professional and fluent manner and ensures they thank the patient. Washes hands	0	1	2

ALLEN's Test:- Elevate the patient's hand and ask them to make a fist for 30 seconds. Put pressure over both the radial and ulnar arteries, occluding them. With the hand still elevated, ask the patient to open their hand (it should appear blanched). Release the ulnar artery and look for the colour returning (within 7 seconds). If the colour does not return in 7 second then the ulnar circulation is insufficient and therefore the radial artery cannot be safely used for the ABG.

Measuring Blood Pressure

		Not done	Adequate	Good
1	Introduces self, explains the procedure, takes consent and confirms identity of patient. Washes hands			
2	Ensures patient is sat comfortably, with no factors that may give a false reading			
3	Exposes arm after ensuring the arm is not painful.			
4	Chooses appropriate cuff size			
5	Places cuff correctly around the arm			
6	Ensures the arm is in the correct position			
7	Ensures that the pressure dial is easily viable and that it is pointing to zero.			
8	Tightens the air valve on the bulb			
9	Palpates the radial artery			
10	Pumps up the cuff until the radial is not palpable			
11	Lets down the pressure rapidly			
12	Palpates the brachial artery			
13	Places the diaphragm of your stethoscope over the brachial pulse			
14	Inflates the cuff to 30mmHg above the one you previously noted			
15	Lets the cuff down at 2-3mmHg/second			
16	Notes the appearance of audible sounds			
17	Notes the disappearance of audible sounds			
18	Records the value correctly			
19	If this attempt is unsuccessful does not forget to let the cuff down fully before having another attempt			
20	Asks examiner if postural hypotension is to be measured (lying and standing blood pressure)			
21	Removes cuff and asks patient whether they want to know the reading. Thanks and reassures patient and washes hands			

1. This is a standard introduction and consent. Do not forget to warn them that the cuff might get a little tight and uncomfortable.
2. Comfort will ensure you do not get a falsely high reading. Obviously if they have an injury to the arm you hope to use for the reading this should be noted early and you should use the other arm. Also explore whether have had any recent stimulants (caffeine, cigarettes) or done any exercise.
3. Remove all clothing from the arm after asking whether this arm is sore at all.
4. Many cuffs now have a guide on them, there tends to be 3 options, a paediatric, normal and large or "thigh" cuff. Use your common sense, depending on the width of the arm.
5. Wind it around the arm in a neat and tight fashion. The lower edge of the cuff should be ideally 2-3 cm above the antecubital fossa .
6. The antecubital fossa should be at heart level, with the arm in slight flexion and well supported (ideally on a table, not by yourself or the patient)

7. You should be able to see the dial easily. If it is not at zero, open the valve and give the cuff a good squeeze.

8. This is to allow you to inflate the cuff
9. This is found on the anterior surface of the wrist laterally
10. Do this as quickly as possible
11. Remembering the value at which the radial pulse disappeared do this as quickly as you can as well.
12. This is found on the medial side of the antecubital fossa
13. You should hear nothing at this stage
14. This will ensure you do not miss a 'silent gap'
15. Do this carefully and steadily. Too slow and you will take too long and cause discomfort to the patient. Too fast and you may miss the points you are looking for.
16. This is the 1st Korotkoff sound and is also the systolic pressure
17. This is the 2nd Korotkoff sound and is also the diastolic pressure. Wait until they have completely gone. Muffling of the sound is not the diastolic.
18. This should be in mmHg with the systolic over the diastolic e.g. 120/80mmHg
19. Also do not forget to warn the patient you are going to have another attempt
20. Postural hypotension may indicate hypovolaemia in the acute situation or autonomic dysfunction in the chronic situation.
21. This should be done swiftly at the end, whilst thanking the patient. Patients may be anxious and/or curious to know the reading but it is wise to ask them if they wish to know before telling them. It is polite to thank the patient. Always wash your hands to reduce the risk of cross-infection.

INTRAVENOUS CANNULATION

		Not Attempted	Attempted inadequate	Attempted adequate
1.	Introduces self, explains the procedure and obtains consent	0	1	2
2.	Identifies patient verbally and using I.D. bracelet	0	1	2
3.	Prepares equipment	0	1	2
4.	Washes hands and wears gloves	0	1	2
5.	Places tourniquet on. Positions arm and selects an appropriate vein	0	1	2
6.	Cleans skin using an alcohol swab and waits 30 seconds or until dry	0	1	2
7.	Holds cannula correctly	0	1	2
8.	Stabilises the vein, passes cannula into the vein at an angle of 15 degrees and observes for flashback	0	1	2
9.	Gently advances cannula after pulling needle back by 2mm	0	1	2
10.	Releases tourniquet	0	1	2
11.	Removes needle whilst maintaining pressure proximal to the cannula and places cap on	0	1	2
12.	Disposes of sharp safely	0	1	2
13.	Secures cannula with a sterile transparent dressing	0	1	2
14.	Assess vein patency using IV normal saline flush	0	1	2
15.	Washes hands	0	1	2
16.	Remains aseptic throughout	0	1	2
17.	Demonstrates a good standard of communication	0	1	2
18.	Thanks the patient	0	1	2

EQUIPMENT: appropriate sized cannula, steret, IV saline flush, 5ml syringe, tourniquet, gloves, gauze/cotton wool, sharps bin.

Venepuncture

		Not Attempted	Attempted inadequate	Attempted adequate
1.	Introduces self to patient, gains consent	0	1	2
2.	Identifies patient verbally/ using ID bracelet and identification on request form	0	1	2
3.	Explains procedure to patients in simple language (not using any jargon)			
4	Assembles appropriate equipment†	0	1	2
5.	Washes hands / wears gloves	0	1	2
6.	Ensures patient is comfortable and that patient's head can be lowered quickly	0	1	2
7.	Applies tourniquet on non dominant arm	0	1	2
8.	Palpates veins to select appropriate site	0	1	2
9.	Cleans the area with alcohol swab and waits for 30 seconds or till dry	0	1	2
10.	Stabilises the vein distally and warns the patient "sharp scratch"	0	1	2
11.	Uses vacutainer system correctly and fills bottle (bevel of needle pointing up)	0	1	2
12.	Places tube into kidney dish	0	1	2
13.	Releases tourniquet	0	1	2
14.	Applies sterile swab to insertion site and removes needle maintaining pressure until bleeding stops	0	1	2
15.	Disposes of needle safely into sharps bin	0	1	2
16.	Completes the procedure in a professional fluent manner	0	1	2
17.	Good aseptic technique throughout	0	1	2
18.	Thanks the patient and ensure bottles are correctly labelled.	0	1	2
19	Washes hands	0	1	2

† EQUIPMENT – Kidney dish containing: Tourniquet, vacutainer needle, a spare needle, alcohol swab, gloves, vacutainer, vacutainer bottles, sterile swab or cotton wool, adhesive dressing tape (or band-aid) and a sharps bin.

Male Catheterisation

		Not Attempted	Attempted inadequate	Attempted adequate
1.	Prepare equipment	0	1	2
2.	Introduce self to patient	0	1	2
3.	Explain procedure and gain consent	0	1	2
4.	Ensures patient privacy, exposes patient and ensures they are comfortable	0	1	2
5.	Wears a plastic apron	0	1	2
6.	Opens pack using aseptic technique	0	1	2
7.	Cleans hands with surgical scrub, dries with a sterile towel, puts on sterile gloves in a 'no-touch' fashion.	0	1	2
8.	Creates a sterile field, using sterile towels so only the penis is visible	0	1	2
9.	Uses left hand to hold the penis with gauze, and with the right hand, cleans the penis with a cotton wool and saline (correct no touch technique)	0	1	2
10.	Disposes of used cotton wool in a yellow bag, away from sterile field	0	1	2
11.	Warns patient and inserts anaesthetic gel into urethra, holding penis vertically up mentions they would wait 3-5 minutes	0	1	2
12.	Warns patient and introduces Catheter gently, guarding against contamination	0	1	2
13.	Checks that the catheter is in the bladder: Observes for urine flow and continues to push a little further.	0	1	2
14.	Inflates balloon with correct amount of normal saline and connects catheter to drainage bag	0	1	2
15.	Replaces foreskin if necessary	0	1	2
16.	Maintains dignity and communicates with the patient throughout	0	1	2
17.	Thanks the patient and washes hands	0	1	2

18.	Documents procedure in the patient's notes (to include indications, catheter size and brief description of the procedure)	0	1	2

Top Tips
- Get patient in the supine position
- Put an absorbent pad under patients buttocks
- To insert the catheter, hold the penis vertically up, gentle insert catheter until you meet resistance. At this stage hold the penis horizontally to pass the catheter past the prostate and into the bladder.
- If it's difficult to pass, ask the patient to give a cough as you pass through the area of resistance.
- If no urine appears initially, press on the patient's bladder.
- If the catheter is not passing easily, do not force it as it may cause urethral trauma. Ask for experienced help.

ROUTINE URINALYSIS

		Not Attempted	Attempted inadequate	Attempted adequate
1.	Identifies correct patient sample using name and one other identifier	0	1	2
2.	Washes hands. Puts on gloves and apron	0	1	2
3.	Checks multistick expiration date	0	1	2
4.	Removes stick (without touching the end)	0	1	2
5.	Dips multistick into urine	0	1	2
6.	Removes stick – taps dry on the side of the specimen to remove excess	0	1	2
7.	Waits for the appropriate length of time (as indicated on the container)	0	1	2
8.	Compares results – reading values without touching container	0	1	2
9.	Disposes of stick safely in a clinical waste bag	0	1	2
10.	Removes gloves and apron	0	1	2
11.	Records results correctly	0	1	2
12.	Does the above in a confident and fluent manner	0	1	2
13	Washes hands			

GENERAL TOPICS

Confirmation of Death and Death Certification

		Not done	Adequate	Good
1	Talks to healthcare professional.	0	1	2
2	Explores immediate details of death	0	1	2
3	Asks for notes and confirm patient identity	0	1	2
4	Observes patient	0	1	2
5	Fixed and dilated pupils	0	1	2
6	No respiratory effort for 3 minutes	0	1	2
7	No pulse for one minute	0	1	2
8	No heart sounds for one minute	0	1	2
9	Other possible tests	0	1	2
10	Washes hands			
11	Documents fully and in detail	0	1	2
12	Liaises with nurses about next of kin	0	1	2
13	Makes sure GP is made aware	0	1	2
14	Consults with senior as to whether a PM is needed	0	1	2
15	Completes death certificate	0	1	2

1. Take a rapid history form the healthcare professional who made you aware of the death. Discover the background to the death and exclude any need to start resuscitation.
2. Ask
    a. When the patient died as far as they are aware
    b. Whether he/she was for resuscitation
    c. What was wrong with them, prior to them passing away.
3. It is vital to make sure that you know who you are dealing with, especially on a busy ward where many patients may be on the end of life pathways.
4. Look at the general appearance and note the absence of respiratory movements
5. This should be to torch light, not natural light. Also be aware that certain drugs can alter the reactivity of pupils
6. Cheyne-Stokes breathing (alternating periods of apnoea and hyper-apnoea) is commonly seen in the period shortly before death, result in apnoeic periods of several minutes in some cases. One should also listen over the lungs and again look for chest movements. Another technique is to hold a reflective surface over the patients nose and mouth to look for fogging.
7. Check both carotids, radials and femorals for a full one minute each. Hypotension can result in the loss of a peripheral pulse, and conditions such a hypothyroidism and hypothermia can slow the pulse rate considerably
8. Be aware that if you hear a "lub – dub" be sure to check it is not your own pulse you can hear! This can be confirmed by taking your own pulse whilst auscultating.
9. Assessing response to pain is not necessary and may be distressing to any relatives who are present. If you are still unsure you may choose to do an ECG or look in the eyes for "railroading" as the blood in the retinal veins separates.
10. Write clearly in the notes including
    a. No vital signs (you may choose to list those above)
    b. Time and date of death
    c. Sign name clearly and include bleep number
    d. Note whether a pacemaker is fitted
    e. It is customary to write "RIP" or similar at the bottom of the notation, but this is up to personal preference.

11. If the family are not present they should be notified as soon as possible. If the family is present at the time of death, you should speak to them to ensure they understand what has happened and to answer any questions they may have. They may be extremely distressed, even if the death was expected.
12. Note the GP name and number and make sure someone, either yourself or a member of staff, informs them
13. This is not always necessary, but if you are unsure, it is always best to ask. Some deaths may need to be reported to the coroner.
14. If appropriate at the time fill in the death certificate
    a. Only if you have seen the patient in the last 14 days
    b. Part 1 is the CAUSE of death e.g. Myocardial Infarction
    c. 1b and 1c are underlying conditions that lead to it e.g. Ischaemic heart disease or Hypertension
    d. Part 2 is for other illnesses that are not directly linked to the death
    e. Do not forget to fill in the counter foil
    f. DO NOT USE ABBREVIATIONS

Dermatological Examination

		Not done	Adequate	Good
1	Introduces self and role	0	1	2
2	Exposes patient adequately, after gaining verbal consent and asking for a chaperone.	0	1	2
3	Asks if there is any pain or discomfort present in any area	0	1	2
4	Begins inspection of the skin condition and notes:	0	1	2
5	Does the patient look ill or well?	0	1	2
6	Colour?	0	1	2
7	Shape?	0	1	2
8	Size?	0	1	2
9	Site?	0	1	2
10	Surface?	0	1	2
11	Edges?	0	1	2
12	In looking specifically and possible malignancy uses the ABCD approach • **A**symmetry • **B**order irregularity • **C**olour irregularity • **D**iameter enlarging	0	1	2
13	Washes hands and palpates the lesion(s)	0	1	2
14	Is it tender? Does it feel warm? Is it hard or soft? Is it firm or fluctuant?	0	1	2
15	Does firm pressure lead to blanching?	0	1	2
16	Does it bleed easily?	0	1	2
17	Examines the rest of the body for further areas especially the elbows, soles of the feet, knees and flexor creases	0	1	2
18	Checks nails and hair	0	1	2
19	Checks pulses if you feel the lesion is an ulcer	0	1	2
20	Are there regional lymph nodes?	0	1	2
21	Covers up, thanks patient and washes hands	0	1	2

1. It is both rapport building an necessary to do this.
2. Ask the patient where they feel the lesions are and expose this area fully. Wipe off any make up or topical preparations that may obscure the true nature of the lesions
3. This will avoid you causing any further undue discomfort to the patient
4. This should be done is a systematic fashion.
5. You must assess these lesions holistically. Are they a sign of a greater infection or pathology? Do you feel there is some systemic going on?
6. Note especially any erythema or if there are a great number of colours present.
7. You must note:
   a. Macule – flat area of discoloration
   b. Plaque – raised area with a flat top
8. In terms of size, note especially
   a. Papule - <1cm of raised/elevated skin
   b. Nodule - >1cm of palpable mass
   c. Is it single or multiple?

9. Note the exact position if a localised lesion. If generalised is it on a flexor or extensor surface? It may be areas of friction or pressure. Is it a warm or sweaty area? Is it possible that it is spread by sexual contact? This applies to genital lesions as well as the lower abdomen and upper thighs. Are the lesions symmetrical or asymmetrical?
10. In terms of the surface, note
    a. Vesicle – blister <5mm
    b. Bulla – blister >5mm
    c. Pustule – blister containing pus
    d. Scale – flaky keratin
    e. Crust – dried exudate
11. Are the edges well demarcated? Irregular or regular?
12. The ABCD approach helps as;
 Non-Suspicious lesions tend to be; Less than 6mm in diameter, with well-defined borders, of a single shade of pigment and generally unchanging over time.

However, suspicious lesions may be; Larger than 6mm across with an irregular notched border with pigment blending into surrounding skin. Their surface may be varied - partly raised, partly flat with numerous colours. There is also frequently a history of change.

13. Do this gently. Do not forget to wash you hands if you have not already done so.
14. These all help in developing one's differential. Certainly pain and warmth can suggest an inflammatory or infectious process.
15. This is part of looking for a meningitic non-blanching rash and should never be omitted.
16. You must see whether the lesion is easily friable? Is it well vascularised? Bleeding is never a good sign!
17. Many patients may not be aware that their dermatological condition is elsewhere on their body. Equally finding the lesions in other site may help your differential. For example, finding lesions on the breast may cause a great deal of concern. But if you can see the rash spreads all the way down the dermatome, you can begin to think in terms of shingles. The pattern of distribution of a rash can be very useful in pointing to a diagnosis.
18. This is both in term of nail and hair changes but also in terms of hair loss and skin changes to the scalp.
19. This will help deciding whether the ulcer is venous or arterial and in relation to possible peripheral vascular disease.
20. This is for infectious or malignant lesions. The three worrying characters of lymph nodes are : Fixed, Non-tender or Large.
21. Do this while maintaining the patient's dignity. It is polite to thank the patient. Always wash your hands to reduce the risk of cross-infection.

Lymph Node Examination

Lymp Node Groups:

Head and Neck	Occipital (base of skull at the back) Post-auricular (behind the ear) Pre-Auricular (in front of the tragus) Tonsillar (below the angle of the mandible) Submandibular (below the mandible) Submental (below the chin)
	Posterior Cervical Chain (Anterior to the Trapezius) Anterior Cervical Chain (Anterior to the SternoCleidoMastoid) Supraclavicular (in the hollow above the clavicle)
Axilla:	Anterior wall Posterior wall Apical Medial (along chest wall)
Groins:	Suprainguinal (above the inguinal ligament) Infrainguinal (below the inguinal ligament) Femoral (medial part of upper thigh)
Popliteal:	Behind the knee

Don't forget to palpate the Spleen in cases of generalised lymphadenopathy.

In cases of localised lymphadenopathy: examine the areas which they drain:

Breast and upper limbs (and upper part of torso) for axillary nodes
Lower limbs, Anus and Scrotum (and lower rorso) for groin nodes,
Head, neck, ENT and thyroid for head and neck nodes.

Oesophageal and Gastric Cancer can cause supcraclavicular nodes to enlarge

Widespread lymphadenopathy should raise the suspicion of a lymphoma

---

Breast History

		Not Attempted	Attempted inadequate	Attempted adequate
1.	Introduces self, explains role and gains consent	0	1	2
2.	Asks what the presenting complaint is	0	1	2
3.	If there is a history of a breast lump, asks: Side Duration Change in size and over what period of time	0	1	2
4.	Asks what symptoms are associated with the lump. Is there: Pain Discomfort Change associated with menstrual cycle	0	1	2
5.	Asks if pain is related to exertion/movement	0	1	2
6.	Asks if there is a nipple discharge. If so asks: Amount Consistency Colour Bloodstained	0	1	2
7.	Asks the patient's age at menarche and menopause (if applicable)	0	1	2
8.	Asks about number of pregnancies and what age the first pregnancy was	0	1	2
9.	Asks about breast feeding	0	1	2
10.	Asks about use of oral contraception and hormonal replacement therapy	0	1	2
11.	Asks about a family history of breast or ovarian cancer	0	1	

1. It is important to introduce yourself, exlain what your role is and obtain verbal consent for the task of taking a history.
2. Most patients present with either a breast lump, breast pain or a nipple discharge.
3. For a breast lump, it is important to note which side it is, how long it has been present and whether there is a change in size. Cancerous lumps usually have a short history and grow progressively in size. Fibroadenomas can fluctuate with the menstrual period.
4. Painful lumps in which the discomfort varies with the menstrual cycle are usually benign.
5. This is to differentiate between musculoskeletal pain and breast pain (mastalgia).
6. Nipple discharge may be an early sign of breast cancer especially if it is bloodstained. Single duct discharge can appear as a bead on expression (it is much better to let the

patient express the discharge). Copious discharge especially if bilateral should point to an endocrine cause.

7-8. Women who under go early menarche and prolonged uninterrupted menstrual periods have a higher risk of breast cancer.

9. Breast feeding reduces the chances of developing breast cancer.

10. OCP and HRT both increase the risk of breast cancer.

11. Family history of breast and ovarian cancer is important as it may identify a familial etiology. If a first degree relative (mother, sister) have had breast cancer at an early age, a full family tree should be drawn to identify whether there is a familial etiology and referral for genetic testing may then be considered. BRCA 1 and 2 are genes associated with familial breast and ovarian cancer.

Breast Examination

		Not Attempted	Attempted inadequate	Attempted adequate
1.	Introduces self, explains role and gains consent	0	1	2
2.	Asks for chaperone and washes hands	0	1	2
3.	Ensures privacy	0	1	2
4.	Adequately exposes patient and positions them correctly.	0	1	2
5.	Inspects breasts and compares with other side with hands on hips and hands behind head	0	1	2
6.	Palpates the breast using good technique using flat of the fingers	0	1	2
7.	Correctly describes any masses	0	1	2
8.	Asks for nipple discharge and asks patient to express discharge	0	1	2
9.	Examines the lymph nodes in axilla	0	1	2
10.	Examines other breast, nipple and axilla	0	1	2
11.	Completes examination by examining the supraclavicular lymph nodes, lung fields, spine and abdomen (if advanced cancer is suspected)	0	1	
12.	Thanks the patient and allows them to dress. Maintains patient dignity throughout	0	1	2
13.	Maintains good communication with patient throughout	0	1	2
14.	Conducts the examination in a fluent professional manner. Washes hands.	0	1	2

1) It is important to introduce yourself (give your full name and role). Explain that you would like to examine their breasts and gain consent.

2) Asking for a chaperone protects you as a doctor from any possible accusations and is a must for both males and females. This can also reassure the patient.

3) Ensuring privacy is important to maintain patient dignity and helps the patient relax.

4) Appropriately expose the patient; ask her to undress to her waist and take off her bra. Position the patient correctly (Sat up for inspection and at 45° for palpation).

5) With the patients arms by their side inspect the breasts. Get down to the level of the patient's breast for the examination to show that you are looking thoroughly. Observe breasts for symmetry, visible masses, erythema, ulceration, peau d'orange (dimpled appearance), radiotherapy marks, scars, and nipple changes/inversion.
Look again at the breasts with the patient's arms above their head and then their arms pressed into hips (tightens pectoralis muscles), this may make any masses more visible depending on the attachment.

6) Enquire whether the breasts are tender. If one breast is tender, start on the opposite breast. With the patient's arm above their head, turning slightly on the contralateral hip. Examine from the mid axillary line to the sternum and from clavicle to bra line. Examine the breast using the flat palmer aspects of fingers to examine all parts of the breast. Maintain flat of fingers parallel to the chest wall, using a circular motion to push into the breast tissue. Using a systematic method, palpate all areas of breast. If the breast is large it may help to use two hands, using one to support the breast tissue.

7) Examine any masses assessing number, shape, size, site (left or right and 1-12'o clock position – distance from nipple in cm), margins and consistency – smooth / rough / firm, skin changes, tenderness, mobile or fixed to skin and pectoralis muscle (ask patient to press hands into hips: mobility is reduced if fixed). Watch for signs of discomfort on their face.

Differentiate between common lumps

Fibroadenoma (breast mouse – highly mobile, rarely painful, smooth, rubbery, small, sometimes multiple)

Carcinoma – rarely painful, irregular, hard, tethering of skin/fixation, nipple changes, bloody discharge, lymphadenopathy. Family history, age 55+, weight loss (advanced tumour metastases can cause backache or jaundice)

Fibroadenosis – cyclical breast pain, smooth, firm, nipple disc white, single/multiple lumps or generally nodular.

8) Note the colour of any discharge. Normal secretions may appear clear or milky. Bloody discharge is a cause for concern and must be investigated further.

9) Examines the lymph node in axillary tail of the breast (in armpit). Palpate all 4 walls and correctly patient's supports arm.

10) Examines other breast

11) Complete the examination by examining the supraclavicular lymph nodes, lung fields for effusion, spine for bony tenderness, abdomen for hepatomegaly. These examinations may indicate the presence of metastases.

12) Cover the patient up. Maintain patient's dignity by not leaving them exposed for longer than necessary.

13) Good communication with patient throughout (Explain what you are doing as you do it).

14) Conduct the examination in a fluent and professional manner. Always wash your hands after each examination.

GYNECOMASTIA:
Genetic **G**ender disorder (Klinefelter)
Young boy (pubertal)*
Neonate*
Estrogen
Cirrhosis/ **C**imetidine/ **Ca C**hannel blockers
Old age*
Marijuana
Alcoholism
Spironolactone
Tumors (**T**esticular & adrenal)
Isoniazid/ **I**nhibition of testosterone
Antineoplastics (**A**lkylating **A**gents)/ **A**ntifungal(ketoconazole)
· * Asterisk indicates physiologic cause.

Preoperative Assessment

		Not Done	Adequate	Good
1	Introduces self and role, whilst confirming correct patient (verbally and wrist band)	0	1	2
2	Confirms operation and left or right side if applicable	0	1	2
3	Clarifies the purpose of the interview	0	1	2
4	Explores patient's feelings on the operation	0	1	2
5	Asks history of presenting complaint	0	1	2
6	Past Medical History	0	1	2
7	Drug History	0	1	2
8	Family History	0	1	2
9	Social History	0	1	2
10	Review of Systems including;	0	1	2
11	Last Menstrual Period (females)	0	1	2
12	Tetanus immunisation	0	1	2
13	Dentures and Crowns	0	1	2
14	GI Tract: Dysphagia, gastro-oesophageal reflux, anorexia or weight loss, change in bowel habit, rectal bleeding.	0	1	2
15	CVS/Resp: Chest Pain, Shortness of breath, Cough, Sputum, Palpitations.	0	1	2
16	Urinary symptoms	0	1	2
17	Fits, Faints and Funny Turns	0	1	2
18	Rashes or joint pain	0	1	2
19	Determines any further patient concerns or expectations	0	1	2
20	Gives opportunity for any questions?	0	1	2
21	Ensures consent has been taken	0	1	2
22	Informs patient of time of operation and given any special instructions	0	1	2
23	Arranges relevant investigations	0	1	2
24	Writes up drugs including thromboprophylaxis	0	1	2
25	Asks patient for any information they would like to give the nurses.	0	1	2
26	Marks side and site of surgery with indelible pen after double checking with notes and patient.	0	1	2
27	Thanks patient and washes hands			

1. Ask the usual confirmatory questions such as Name or Date of Birth
2. Use an open question such as, "I understand you are coming in for an operation on ...., is that correct?"
3. Make it clear that this interview is to minimise any risks before, during or after the operation. Reassure the patient at this stage that this interview would be a good time to ask any questions and make the team aware of any concerns or worries.
4. Ask open questions. You should actively encourage the patient to contribute and responds well to any concerns they might have, exploring them as needed. The

candidate should be sensitive to the patient's non-verbal or verbal cues; hand wringing, appearing nervous, ad phrases such as "so what are the risks again?"

5. This should be brief and concise. No more than a few sentences.
6. This should be as complete as possible and include;
   a. Any previous medical problems or previous admission
   b. Past operations +/- complications
   c. Previous anaesthetic history
   d. Chronic diseases, explicitly *HASH CREDIT*
      i. **H**ypertension
      ii. **A**sthma/COPD
      iii. **S**ickle cell
      iv. **H**IV and **H**ep
      v. **C**VA
      vi. **R**heumatic fever
      vii. **E**pilepsy
      viii. **D**iabetes
      ix. **I**schaemic Heart Disease
      x. **T**B
7. This should also be as complete as possible, asking specifically about *CASES* and allergies to *AAA*
      i. **C**ontraceptives
      ii. **A**nticoagulants
      iii. **S**teroids
      iv. **E**thanol
      v. **S**moking
   b. **A**naesthetics
   c. **A**ntibiotics
   d. **A**pplications (eg elastoplasts, iodine etc)
8. Ask about DVT, PE and other clotting or bleeding problems as well as family history of allergies, especially to anaesthetic
9. Social support, living conditions, occupation, mobility, any dependants.
10. – 18. These all affect the pre and post operative risks and complications.
19. One should make a careful effort to seek and address and specific needs the patient might have.
20. You can also use this juncture to summarise what has been elicited so far.
21. If not, reassure that it will be done, in full before the procedure.
22. Only if this information is available to you, i.e. 2pm and nil by mouth from breakfast.
23. Preoperative investigations should include; FBC +/- blood film, Clotting, Group and Save +/- crossmatch, U&E, LFT, ECG, CXR and a blood sugar
24. You must consider appropriate drugs; Fluids, analgesia, anticoagulation, antibiotics
25. The date and time of the operation, when to make nil by mouth, to give analgesia, monitor vital signs, to keep a fluid balance chart and to inform any specialist nurses that may need to be involved.
26. It is polite to thank the patient. Always wash your hands to reduce the risk of cross-infection.

Examination of an Ulcer

		Not Attempted	Attempted inadequate	Attempted adequate
1.	Introduces self, explains role and gains consent	0	1	2
2.	Asks the patient where the ulcer is present. Asks for a chaperone if appropriate.	0	1	2
3.	Ensures privacy	0	1	2
4.	Adequately exposes the ulcer and positions it in good light. Washes hands and wears sterile gloves before examination	0	1	2
5.	Inspects ulcer commenting on: Smell Site Size Shape Edge Floor Pigmentation Discharge Surrounding skin or mucosa	0	1	2
6.	Asks if it is tender and palpates ulcer gently bimanually with both index fingers. Looks for fixity to underlying structures, tenderness and bleeding.	0	1	2
7.	Palpates the skin around the ulcer	0	1	2
8.	Palpates the regional lymph nodes draining the ulcer	0	1	2
9.	Palpates the arterial supply to the area of the ulcer	0	1	2
10.	If ulcer is on the lower leg, stands patient and looks for varicose veins	0	1	2
11.	If ulcer is in the peri-anal area, asks to perform a digital rectal examination			
12.	Thanks the patient and allows them to dress. Maintains patient dignity throughout	0	1	2
13.	Maintains good communication with patient throughout	0	1	2
14.	Conducts the examination in a fluent professional manner. Thanks patient and washes hands	0	1	2

1) It is important to introduce yourself (give your full name and role). Explain that you would like to examine them and gain consent.

2) Ask the patient where the ulcer is located. Asking for a chaperone protects you as a doctor from any possible accusations and is a must for both males and females. This can also reassure the patient.

3) Ensuring privacy is important to maintain patient dignity and helps the patient relax.

4) Appropriately expose the ulcer and ensure there is good light. For mouth ulcers, a torch will be required. Remove any dressings or plasters and always wash your hands and wear sterile gloves before touching the ulcer.

5) A foul smell indicates an anaerobic infection of the ulcer. 95% of rodent ulcers (basal cell carcinomas) occur on the upper part of the face. Carcinomas typically affect the lower lip. Size is important especially in the length of the history. Indolent lonstanding ulcers are often vascular in etiology and rapidly growing ones indicate malignancy or infection. Basal Cell Cancers are usually circular. Venous ulcers usually occur on the medial aspect of the lower leg and are oval in shape. A rodent ulcer has a rolled edge, a malignant ulcer has a raised and everted edge. The floor of the ulcer is the visible base and may be filled with blood clot or slough. Pigmented ulcers may indicate A purulent discharge indicates an active infection. The surrounding skin of a venous ulcer is pigmented and thickened while in arterial ulcers it is hairless and thin.

6) Enquire whether the ulcer is tender. Palpate gently bimanually with both index fingers. Fixity to deeper structures and may indicate invasion of deeper layers by a malignant ulcer which may also bleed easily.

7) Look for thickening or attenuation.

8) This is essential as palpable regional lymph nodes indicate their involvement in the pathological process.

9) This will rule out an arterial ulcer

10) Typicall, these ulcers are on the medial aspect of the lower leg (above the ankle) and are surrounded by pigmented thickened skin. Standing may fill the varicosities and make them obvious.

11) Peir-anal ulcers may be simple fissures, squamous cancers or caused by Crohn's disease.

12) Thank the patient and ask them to re-dress if required.

13) Good communication with patient throughout (Explain what you are doing as you do it).

14) Conduct the examination in a fluent and professional manner. Always wash your hands after each examination.

Types of Ulcer

VAN:
Venous/ **V**asculitic
Arterial
Neuropathic

EXAMINATION OF A LUMP

		Not Attempted	Attempted inadequate	Attempted adequate
1.	Introduces self, explains role and gains consent	0	1	2
2.	Asks the patient where the lump is present. Asks for a chaperone if appropriate. Ensures privacy.	0	1	2
3.	Adequately exposes the lump and positions it in good light. Washes hands before examination	0	1	2
4.	Inspects lump commenting on: Site Size Shape Overlying skin	0	1	2
5.	Asks if it is tender and palpates lump gently bimanually with both index fingers. Comments on: Tenderness, temperature. Size Consistency Fluctuation Pulsatility Fixity to skin Fixity to underlying structures Surrounding skin	0	1	2
6.	Palpates the regional lymph nodes draining the lump	0	1	2
7.	Thanks the patient and allows them to dress. Maintains patient dignity throughout. Washes hands.	0	1	2

1. It is important to introduce yourself, explain your role and task and gain verbal consent.
2. Ask the patient where the lump is present and if this means exposing the patient, it is best to ask for a chaperone first.
3. Expose the area where the lump is present and always wash your hands before examining it.
4. Comment on its site, size, shape and what the overlying skin is like (e.g., ulcerated, discoloured, inflamed).
5. Always ask about tenderness and be very careful not to hurt the patient if they say it is tender. Assess whether it is an inflammatory or infective lesion (by checking temperature, and tenderness). Assess the size, consistency, fluctuation (3 finger method- put the index and middle fingers of your left hand at the edges of the lump and press with tip of the index finger of the right hand. If there is fluid in the lump, you will feel it with your left hand). Check pulsatility again with index and middle fingers of one hand. Fixity to skin is assessed by pinching the skin over the lump, if you can pinch it, it is not fixed to the skin (and thus not arising from it either). Fixity to deeper structures is assessed by tensing the underlying muscle, if this reduces mobility of the lump, it is fixed to the underlying muscle. Feel the surrounding skin for induration or cellulitis.

6. Always palpate the regional lymph nodes (see Top-Tips on lymph node examination)
7. It is polite to thank the patient. Always wash your hands to reduce the risk of cross-infection.

Top Tips

Looking at Fracture X-rays

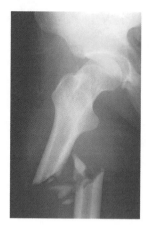

As with all types of x-ray film you should have a 'system' for looking at fractures where you expect you may find an abnormality. Having a system that you can repeat easily means you are less likely to miss something and also allows you to easily and smoothly present your findings in the exam setting. It is best to do a directed search of the film rather than simply gazing at the film. An abnormality will not always be glaringly obvious. Therefore, it is best to look for abnormalities and to have a planned search in mind. Your eye gaze should scan all portions of the film, in an orderly fashion.

More importantly, the identification and proper classification of fractures is vital in determining the subsequent treatment and long term management of the patient.

Before looking at the x-ray itself there are always certain things you should check and comment on
- Name
- Age
- Gender
- Indication for x-ray (if available)
- Type of x-ray (eg "this is an AP film of the...)

Once you have looked at these, you can present them in a simple and concise way, such as: "This is an AP and lateral film of Mr X's femur, born 31/02/1986 and was taken after he was involved in a head-on RTA".

After this one can use the ATLS system for looking at any trauma x-ray

AABC'S

A – Adequacy
A – Alignment
B – Bones
C – Cartilage
S – Soft tissues

Adequacy

On a high quality radiograph you should be able to see the entire bone you wish to view, ideally including the joint above and joint below where you feel the fracture is. Equally the film should be clear and not too "white" or too "dark". If this is the case, then an

228

insufficient number of x-rays have passed through the patient to reach the x-ray film. As a result the film will look 'whiter' leading to potential 'overcalling' of pathology. Similarly, if the film appears too 'black', then too many xrays have resulted in overexposure of the x-ray film. This 'blackness' results in pathology being less conspicuous and may lead to 'undercalling'.

Alignment

The reason we tend to get two views when x-raying a fracture is so we can comment on alignment. We must remember that fractures happen in 3 dimensions and as such we must be able to see the alignment at the fracture site. One must describe whether the fracture fragments are displaced or in their normal anatomical position. If the bones fragments aren't in the right place, they need to be reduced or placed back into their normal alignment. The description can simply be done in terms of medial/lateral/anterior/posterior, such as "The most proximal segment of the fracture is anteriorly displaced." The terms 'valgus' and 'varus'

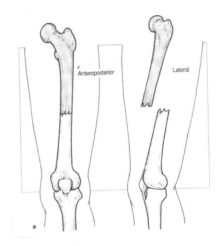

describe the alignment between two anatomical segments. Draw a line through the long axis of the proximal segment and draw another line to illustrate the long axis the distal segment. Compare the two lines, focusing on the alignment of the distal segment *with respect to the proximal segment*. In a **varus** alignment, the distal segment deviates medially with respect to the proximal segment. In a **valgus** alignment, the distal segment deviates laterally with respect to the proximal segment.

Bones

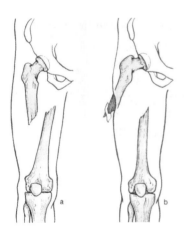

This is, with fractures at least, where the bulk of the work is.

1. Begin by commenting on whether the fracture is open or closed. If the skin over the break is disrupted, even in the slightest, then an open fracture exists. It does not matter on the degree, (cut, torn, or abraded), but if the skin's integrity is damaged, the infection risk is increased. These injuries need to be cleaned out aggressively and may require cleaning and debridement in theatres to do the job effectively. Air in the soft tissues or the fracture site is a useful sign.

2. You then need to comment on the type of fracture you can see.

Oblique - a fracture which goes at an angle to the axis

Comminuted - a fracture of many relatively small fragments

Spiral - a fracture which runs around the axis of the bone

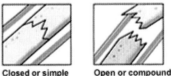

Closed or simple fracture.   Open or compound fracture.

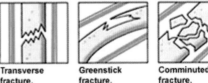

Transverse fracture.   Greenstick fracture.   Comminuted fracture.

There are different sub-types of fracture that you should be able to identify and comment on:

Articular. a fracture of the joint surface of a bone; called also joint fracture.	**Fissured** a crack extending from a surface into, but not through, a long bone.
Avulsion. an indirect fracture caused by avulsion or pull of a ligament.	**Greenstick**. fracture in which one side of a bone is broken, the other being bent (usually in babies/young children)
Axial compression. fracture of a vertebra by excessive vertical force, so that pieces of it move out in horizontal directions, often injuring the spinal cord; it usually occurs in the thoracic or lumbar region as a result of flexion.	**Hairline** a fracture that appears in the radiograph as a fine hairlike line, the segments of bone not being separated; sometimes seen in fractures of the skull
Basal neck. fracture of the neck of the femur at its junction with the trochanteric region.	**Intra-articular**. a fracture of the articular surface of a bone.
Bennett's Fracture: Fracture dislocation of the first metacarpal bone. Caused by a blow to the point of the thumb	**Intracapsular**. fracture within the capsule of a joint.
	Mallet Finger: Avulsion of a flake of bone to which the long extensor tendon is attached
Boxer's. fracture of the metacarpal neck with volar displacement of the metacarpal head caused by striking a hard object with the closed fist.	**Pathological**. one due to weakening of the bone structure by pathologic processes, such as neoplasia, osteomalacia, osteomyelitis, and other diseases.
Bursting. a comminuted fracture of the distal phalanx; called also tuft f.	**Periarticular**. a fracture extending close to, but not into, a joint.
Butterfly. a comminuted fracture in which there are two fragments on each side of a main fragment, resembling the wings of a butterfly.	**Pott's** fracture of the lower part of the fibula, with serious injury of the lower tibial articulation, usually a chipping off of a portion of the medial malleolus, or rupture of the medial ligament.
Colles'. fracture of the lower end of the radius in which the lower fragment is displaced posteriorly. A reverse Colles' fracture or **Smith's fracture** is one in which the lower fragment is displaced anteriorly.	**Salter-Harris**. an epiphyseal fracture in children that involves the epiphyseal growth plate. (*see Salter Harris Definition later*)
Compression. one produced by compression, as of a vertebra (also called a crush fracture)	**Wedge-compression**. compression fracture of only the anterior part of a vertebra, leaving a wedge-shaped vertebra.
Epiphyseal. fracture at the point of union of an epiphysis with the shaft of a bone.	
Extracapsular. a fracture of the head of humerus or femur outside of the capsule of the joint.	

Salter Harris Fractures

These are a fracture type you should always be aware of in children, and by children this should include anyone who you feel is still growing. There are 5 types;

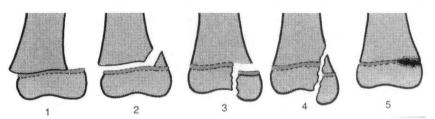

1. Epiphyseal slip only
2. Fracture through the epiphyseal plate with a triangular fragment of shaft left attached to the epiphysis
3. Fracture through the epiphysis extending to the epiphyseal plate
4. Fracture through the epiphysis and shaft crossing the epiphyseal plate
5. Obliteration of the epiphyseal plate

It is a simple fact there are enough different fractures to write an entire book on. Pelvic fractures, spinal fractures, hip fractures and so on. Thus it is important to be aware of the more common type one might see. However, using the information above a simple, concise summary of a fracture can be delivered,

"There is a closed spiral fracture of the left femur noted in the proximal 1/3 of the bone, in line with the mechanism of injury reported by the patient."

Cartilage

Cartilage is an often over looked aspect of fracture inspection. Damage to cartilage can easily occur with a traumatic fracture. This can then go on to cause subsequent arthritic changes and quite a great deal of pain for the patient.

Soft Tissues

- These can be to:
    - Blood Vessels
    - Nerves
    - Muscle
    - Skin
    - Viscera

Any traumatic injury can cause an injury to soft tissue. The force required to break a bone is normally large enough to cause damage in itself, but the jagged and often sharp edges of a fractured bone are perfectly capable of damages surrounding structures.

It is possible to see this damage on an x-ray, as soft tissues tend to appear in shades of grey, swellings and haematomas can sometimes be seen.

Blood vessels can be damaged by;

- Complete division
- Stretching
- Spasm
- soft tissue damage to the wall

Nerves can suffer;

- Neurapraxia – transient loss of function caused by outside pressure.
- Axonotmesis – loss of function due to more severe compression but without the loss of continuity of the neurone.
- Neurotmesis – Division of the nerve, no neural continuity.

Muscle can be damaged in four ways
- Crushing
- Laceration
- Ischaemia
- Ectopic Ossification

Skin can suffer:
- Direct Trauma
- Stretching
- Degloving
And finally…

It is common for an examiner to ask how long you think this injury will take to heal. A good rule of thumb is

"Bones join in 8 weeks, double for the lower limb, half for children."

Images courtesy of Google Image Search – Fracture(s)

Top Tips

Assessment of the Acutely Ill Patient

- Don't panic! There are very few emergencies to which you have to run
- Acutely ill patients do not usually arrive with a diagnostic label, so treating problems as you find them, while simultaneously looking for a cause, is often necessary
- Taking your time and performing a systematic (ABCDE) assessment is the only way to get anywhere
- Don't forget to ask for help

Primary Survey

This is where you eyeball the patient, decide whether they need immediate simultaneous assessment and resuscitation along ABCD lines, or whether the usual approach of careful history taking and examination, followed by investigations, is more appropriate. If your 'eyeball test' suggests a problem, the primary survey involves assessment of airway, breathing, circulation and disability, addressing problems as you find them. You will still need to do a full history and examination, but these may follow the resuscitation phase.

Airway with cervical spine control

Look for:
- Evidence of airway obstruction
- Inadequate airway reflexes to protect an airway (decreased conscious level)

Assessment:
- Can the patient talk normally? (If so, the airway is patent)
- Stridor / gurgling / snoring (partial airway obstruction)
- Look at the oxygen mask – is it misting and demisting with respiration?
- Look in mouth for foreign bodies etc
- Feel for breath

Actions:
- Apply Oxygen
- If evidence of actual or potential airway obstruction – get help urgently
- Check for obvious foreign bodies in airway
- Consider gentle suctioning of mouth if secretions or vomit are present

If airway obstruction associated with decreased conscious level:
- Airway manoeuvres (chin lift, jaw thrust)
- Naso- or oro-pharyngeal airways
- Recovery position (unless suspected spinal injury)
- Reverse obvious causes (eg opioid toxicity)

Tips:
- A fall in O_2 saturation is a late sign in airway obstruction

- Remember the chest will still move and work of breathing may be increased dramatically.
- In patients with a tracheostomy tube in place with the cuff inflated, breathing through the mouth/nose is not possible. A blocked tracheostomy tube should be treated with attempted suctioning or, if unsuccessful, deflation of the cuff allowing breathing through the mouth past the tracheostomy.

Breathing
- Look for:
    - Obvious distress
    - Cyanosis
    - Use of accessory muscles
    - Respiratory rate (This is the single most useful marker of critical illness)
- Feel for:
    - Tracheal tug/deviation
    - Chest wall movement + expansion
- Listen for:
    - Air entry/breath sounds
    - Added sounds
- Check:
    - Oxygen Saturations (aim for >92% in most patients)

Causes of severe breathing problems:
There are only a few things that commonly cause life-threatening breathing problems:
- Pneumonia
- Atelectasis
- Bronchospasm (usually asthma or COPD)
- Pulmonary oedema
- Pulmonary embolus
- Pneumothorax

Tips:
- O_2 Saturation < 95% in a previously healthy patient is not normal
- Hypoxia kills more quickly that hypercarbia, so if hypoxic, give oxygen.
- Don't be fooled by apparently normal O_2 saturations or PaO_2 if high concentrations of oxygen are required
- Hypercapnia usually results from respiratory muscle fatigue due to increased work of breathing. The treatment is ventilatory support, not reduction of oxygen delivery
- Patients may become dangerously hypercapnic and acidotic before the SpO_2 falls, so regular blood gases are essential in unwell patients.
- Not everyone with tachypnoea has a primary respiratory problem, it can be secondary to a metabolic acidosis or a CNS problem
- Remember that adequate cardiac output and haemoglobin concentration are required for oxygen delivery to the tissues

Circulation
- Look for:
    - Colour – pale? Grey? Mottled?
    - JVP
- Listen for:
    - Heart sounds
- Feel for:
    - Peripheries warm or cool
    - Capillary refill time (central over bony prominence eg sternum)
    - Central pulse – rate, volume, regular
    - Oedema
    - Peripheral pulses
- Check:
    - BP
    - ECG rhythm
    - Urine output (useful sign of poor perfusion in shock)

Circulatory problems:
- Shock is a failure to adequately perfuse organs, not just hypotension
- Think of the cardiovascular system as plumbing:

Type of shock	Problem	Typical causes	Peripheries	Pulses
Hypovolaemic	Not enough fluid	Bleeding, dehydration	Cold, ↑CRT*	Weak, fast
Cardiogenic	Pump failure	Arrhythmia, MI, cardiomyopathy	Cold, ↑CRT*	Weak, fast
Obstructive	Blocked pipes	Pulmonary embolus, cardiac tamponade, tension pneumothorax	Cold, ↑CRT*	Weak, fast
Distributive	Dilated, leaky pipes	Sepsis, anaphylaxis	Warm, CRT normal* OR Cold, ↑CRT*	Bounding, fast OR Weak, fast
Neurogenic	Dilated pipes	Spinal cord injury	Warm, CRT normal*	Bounding, slow

*Normal capillary refill time is < 2 seconds

Tips:
- Hypotension may be a late sign of shock in young patients
- Check baseline blood pressure: 110/50 mmHg may be normal for some patients, but grossly hypotensive for others
- Fluid resuscitation is the first-line treatment for shock - unless there is *obvious* pulmonary oedema, a *fluid challenge* is worthwhile
- A fluid challenge consists of rapid infusion of a small volume of fluid (eg 250 mls Hartmann's solution) with *assessment of response* – peripheral temperature, HR, BP, and urine output. This is the safest way to give fluid resuscitation and allows titration to effect and less guesswork.
- Do not just increase the maintenance fluids and walk away!
- In cardiogenic shock, fluids may still be required but should be given cautiously, and the mainstay of management is to treat any immediate cause eg arrhythmia or ischaemia, with inotropes as needed (in a critical care setting).
- Never use hypotonic fluids e.g. 5% dextrose for resuscitation purposes.
- If the patient is bleeding and hypotensive, use blood, ideally cross-matched, but type-specific or O Rhesus negative blood can be given in an emergency

Disability

This should be a quick neurological screen - the time to do a full assessment is later:
Ask the questions:

- Is there a decreased conscious level such that the airway is at risk?
- Is there evidence of an immediately remediable cause (eg seizure, hypoglycaemia, opioid toxicity)?
- Is there evidence of a new focal neurological deficit?

Assessment

- AVPU score – Alert / Responsive to Voice / Responsive to Pain / Unresponsive
- GCS (E,M,V)
- Pupils – equal & reactive?
- Seizure activity
- Movement of all limbs?
- Check capillary blood glucose (DEFG – don't ever forget glucose)

Tips

- Deterioration in conscious level may have a primary neurological cause, or may be a response to other pathology eg shock and inadequate cerebral perfusion
- Airway protection may be indicated if conscious level is decreased (GCS <8 or 'P' or 'U' on the AVPU scale are typically regarded as indications for intubation)
- If there is new onset focal neurology, ask whether it may be due to intracranial haemorrhage or other remediable cause where time is of the essence
- Confusion / agitation can be a manifestation of hypoxia / shock / hypoglycaemia / lots of other things for which sedation is not the treatment.
- Do not sedate confused patients until you have identified and treated organic causes as far as possible
- Prevention of secondary brain injury due to hypoxia, hypercapnia, hyperglycaemia and hyperthermia is the most important thing you can do for many patients with brain injury.

Secondary Assessment

- History
- Abdominal, neurological or other examination as indicated
- Input / output chart – consider urinary catheter and hourly urometry
- Review medications
- CXR / ECG / ABG / Blood tests / Other investigations as required
- ABG analysis is not just for diagnosing respiratory failure – it gives information on perfusion and lots of other useful things
- Find out normal state – ask nurses / check notes / call relative
- Are you competent to deal with this patient by yourself or should you ask for help?
- Does the patient have sufficient reversible pathology to make them a candidate for critical care? If so, *refer early*.

Specific Management of Some Common Emergencies

1. Cardiac Arrest

Basic Life Support (BLS):

Call for Help

A: Head tilt + chin lift/jaw thrust. Clear mouth.

B: Breathing? If so, place in recovery position and continue assessment

If not, check pulse

C: Pulse?   If not present, give 30 chest compressions at 100/minute, per 2 breaths.

If present, treat as respiratory arrest

Advanced Life Support (ALS):

1. If witnessed, monitored VT or VF arrest - give precordial thump.

2. Basic Life Support until defibrillator arrives

3. Attach defibrillator / monitor and assess rhythm

4. **VF or pulseless VT**: DC Shock 150 joules (biphasic); immediately restart CPR for 2 minutes; reassess rhythm & pulse; reshock 150 joules.

5. **Asystole or PEA**: 2 minutes CPR; reassess rhythm & pulse.

6. During CPR: correct reversible causes, intubate, obtain IV access, give 1mg IV Adrenaline every 4 minutes

7. If Asystole or PEA with Rate < 60, Atropine 3mg.

8. Consider amiodarone and magnesium, pacing, bicarbonate

Reversible causes (4Hs + 4Ts):

*   Hypoxia
    Hypovolaemia
    Hypokalaemia, hyperkalaemia
    Hypothermia

*   Tension pneumothorax
    Tamponade
    Toxic/therapeutic disturbance
    Thromboembolic / mechanical obstruction

2. Respiratory Arrest

*   Call for help

*   Open airway – position, manoeuvres, adjuncts

*   Bag-valve-mask ventilation with supplementary oxygen

*   Look for reversible causes eg drug toxicity

*   Consider LMA insertion

*   Definitive airway may be required ie intubation

3. Angina

Monitoring /Morphine

Oxygen

Nitrates

Aspirin

4. Myocardial Infarction

- ABC
- O_2 (high flow)
- ECG Monitor
- IV Access
- Check FBP, U+E, Glucose, Lipids

- Aspirin 300mg
- Morphine (5-10mg IV) or Diamorphine (2-5mg IV) + Antiemetic eg Metoclopramide
- GTN spray or Buccal Suscard (caution if hypotensive)
- Beta-blocker titrated to HR <70 (eg. metoprolol 5-15mg IV, unless asthma or LVF)

- Call for help
- Consider clopidogrel 300mg
- Consider thrombolytic therapy (eg Reteplase) or primary percutaneous intervention

- CXR
- Treat hypertension, heart failure, arrhythmias, diabetes, hypercholesterolaemia Check Troponin 6-12 hours post event
- DVT Prophylaxis
- Secondary prevention

Contraindications to Thrombolytic Therapy (Relative and Absolute)

- Recent trauma / surgery
- Bleeding disorder
- Pregnancy
- Head injury
- Previous haemorrhagic CVA
- CVA within 6 months
- Brain tumour
- Active peptic ulcer
- Active bleeding (not menstruation)
- Prolonged CPR
- Warfarin therapy

5. Pulmonary Oedema

- ABCD assessment
- Oxygen
- IV access
- ABG / CXR / ECG
- Treat myocardial ischaemia with nitrates / aspirin / thrombolytics as required
- Furosemide 20-80mg IV as required
- Nitrates (GTN spray sublingual or IV infusion) unless hypotensive
- Consider small dose of opioid (eg morphine 2.5mg)
- CPAP
- Inotropes as required (in critical care setting)

6. Tachyarrhythmia

- ABCD
- Oxygen
- IV access
- Check FBP, U+E, Calcium, Magnesium
- 12-lead ECG or rhythm strip

If unstable (hypotension, chest pain, severe dyspnoea, syncope):

- DC cardioversion -150J biphasic under GA or sedation
- If unsuccessful after 3 attempts, give amiodarone 300mg over 10-20minutes and repeat DC shock

If stable and narrow complex

- Assess rhythm: AF- rate control with Beta blocker, digoxin or amiodarone
- If regular (SVT), attempt vagal manoeuvres and adenosine 6mg, 12mg, 12mg
- If unsuccessful – consider beta blocker, verapamil or amiodarone

If stable and broad complex

- Assess rhythm: VT - amiodarone 300mg over 20-60mins, then 900mg over 24 hours
- Torsade de Pointes- magnesium 2g over 10mins
- SVT with BBB – treat as SVT
- AF with aberrant conduction – treat as AF

7. Bradyarrhythmia

ABCD

Oxygen

IV access

ECG

Unstable? (hypotension, rate <40, heart failure, syncope, ventricular arrhythmias):

- Atropine 500 mcg IV. Repeat up to max 3mg
- Consider adrenaline 2-10 mcg/kg/min or other chronotropic agent
- Transcutaneous pacing
- Consider transvenous pacing

Stable?

- Assess risk of asystole
- High risk if:
    - Recent episode of asystole
    - Mobitz Type 2 AV block
    - Complete heart block with broad QRS
    - Ventricular pause > 3sec
- If any of these features are present, treat as unstable

8. Pulmonary Embolus

- ABCD assessment
- Oxygen
- Fluid challenge if shocked
- LMW Heparin eg Enoxaparin 1.5mg/kg SC OD or Heparin infusion if shocked
- ABG / CXR / ECG
- Bedside Echocardiography if unstable
- If shocked- consider thrombolysis or surgical embolectomy
- TED stockings
- VQ scan or CT Pulmonary Angiography to confirm diagnosis

9. Acute Severe Asthma

Signs of severe attack (any one of):

- Inability to complete sentences in one breath
- Resp rate > 25/minute
- Pulse > 110/minute
- Peak flow 33-50% of predicted or best

Signs of Life-threatening attack (any one of):

- Peak flow < 33% of predicted or best
- Silent chest, cyanosis, poor respiratory effort
- Bradycardia or Hypotension
- Exhaustion, confusion, or coma
- Normal or high $PaCO_2$
- PaO_2 < 8kPa, SpO_2 <92%, cyanosis

Treatment:

- Sit patient up
- High flow O_2
- Salbutamol nebuliser (5mg) with O2. Repeat continuously if needed.
- Hydrocortisone (200mg IV)
- Ipratropium Bromide (500mcg) nebuliser 6 hourly
- Consider Magnesium infusion, salbutamol or aminophylline infusion
- CXR - exclude pneumothorax / pneumonia
- Consider antibiotics if evidence of infection
- Consider ITU referral early

10. Anaphylaxis

Symptoms & signs:

- Skin: Itching, Erythema, Urticaria, Oedema.
- Breathing: wheeze, tongue swelling, laryngeal obstruction, stridor.
- Cardiovascular: tachycardia, hypotension

Management:

- Stop likely precipitants
- Assess ABCD
- High-flow Oxygen
- If respiratory obstruction present – call anaesthetist
- IV access
- If hypotensive or airway obstruction - Adrenaline IM, 0.5ml of 1:1000 (=0.5mg), repeat each 5 minutes if needed
- Chlorphenirimine (Piriton) 10mg IV
- Hydrocortisone 200mg IV
- IV fluid resuscitation with saline or colloid (eg 500ml stat). Be guided by response to successive fluid challenges
- If wheeze, treat as for asthma.
- Consider critical care referral

11. Diabetic Ketoacidosis

Dehydration is more life threatening than any hyperglycaemia.

Signs & symptoms:

Polyuria, lethargy, hyperventilation, ketotic breath, dehydration, vomiting, abdominal cramp, coma.

Management:

- ABCD assessment and treatment.
- Expect tachypnoea and signs of dehydration +/- shock
- IV fluids (Typical regime: 0.9% Saline 1 litre stat, 1L over 1hr, 1L over 2hr, 1L over 4hr. Switch to 5% dextrose when glucose<15mmol/L). Be guided by local protocol and response.
- Plasma glucose. If > 20mmol/L give 10 units soluble insulin (actrapid) IV. Tests: Lab glucose, U+E and PO_4^{3-}, HCO_3^-, osmolality, blood gases, FBP, CRP, blood culture, urinary ketones & MSU.
- Insulin IV sliding scale with hourly blood glucose tests.
- Potassium replacement – be guided by regular U+E measurement
- Consider NG Tube if nausea / vomiting
- Consider antibiotics if infective precipitant

12. Acute GI bleed and Shock

- Assess ABCD
- Protect airway if required. Nil by mouth.
- High-flow O_2
- 2 large bore IV cannulae.
- Draw bloods (Group and crossmatch, FBP, U+E, LFT, glucose, clotting screen).
- Rapid IV colloids or isotonic crystalloid bolus eg Hartmann's solution
- If still shocked: group specific or O negative blood until cross-matched blood available. (If not shocked, slow IV fluids to keep lines open).
- Correct coagulopathy: Vit K, FFP, platelets and cryoprecipitate as required guided by coagulation screen results
- NG tube
- Monitor vitals each 15 minutes, and urine output (>30ml/hr)
- Keep warm – warmed IV fluids, forced air blanket
- Refer to surgeon or gastroenterologist for endoscopy
- High dose Proton Pump Inhibitor
- Terlipressin if suspected variceal bleeding
- Sengstaken tube may be a useful holding measure for variceal bleeding

13. Septic Shock

- ABCD assessment
- High-flow oxygen
- 2 wide bore IV cannulae
- Fluid challenge (eg 500mls Hartmann's solution over 15 minutes) with reassessment and repeat as required
- Urinary catheter and hourly urometry
- Blood, urine, sputum, and other cultures as required
- IV antibiotics according to likely source and local policy
    - Broad spectrum eg Piperacillin / Tazobactam if source unknown
- Further investigation to identify source of sepsis (eg cultures and imaging)
- If shocked despite fluid resuscitation, consider early critical care referral

14. Status epilepticus

- ABCD with particular emphasis on airway patency due to reduced conscious level
- High flow oxygen
- IV access
- Check blood glucose and treat hypoglycaemia
- Lorazepam 2-4mg. Repeat after 5 mins if ongoing seizure activity
- Phenytoin 18mg/kg over 20 mins (ECG monitoring essential)
- If still fitting, contact anaesthetist – likely to need anaesthesia with thiopentone
- Treat electrolyte abnormalities and precipitating cause eg infection, raised ICP

15. Hyperkalaemia

- Usually treat if K+ > 6.0mmol/l and ECG changes or >6.5mmol/l without ECG changes
- Typical ECG changes: tall peaked T waves, wide QRS complexes, sine waves, VT, VF

Actions:

- ECG monitoring
- Check result (Correct patient, haemolysis present, etc)
- 12-lead ECG
- 10mls Calcium carbonate 10% (stabilises cell membrane for about 20 minutes)
- 10 units Actrapid insulin with 50mls 50% dextrose
- Repeat sample
- Nebulised Salbutamol 5mg (can be given continuously if needed)
- Consider oral calcium resonium resin
- Consider sodium bicarbonate if coexistent metabolic acidosis

Scenarios

See how you would handle some real life situations. How much have you learnt from your experiences and reading the summary above?

For each case, discuss your assessment and management – you may have enough information already to tell you what action to take. It's not about the diagnosis, it's about assessing and managing ABCDs. For exams, a good way to phrase your answer is:

"I would go immediately to see the patient and assess airway, breathing, circulation and disability, give oxygen and obtain IV access before taking a full history and examination. In this case, the patient's airway…"

---

1. You are called to see a 38-year old patient who has been admitted following an overdose of diazepam and alcohol. His GCS was 11 on admission, but is now 8. The nurses are concerned that he is making loud snoring noises and his oxygen saturations are 88% on room air.

---

2. You are asked to admit a 45-year old asthmatic patient, who is complaining of chest tightness and breathlessness. She has been given a 5mg salbutamol nebuliser, which helped a little. Her SpO2 is 95% but she is wheezy and unable to complete sentences due to breathlessness and has a respiratory rate of 32 / min.

---

3. You are called to see Mrs Jones (73) in the fractures ward where she is day 1 following left hip hemiarthroplasty. Her current medications include furosemide, rampiril, and spironolactone tablets, and salbutamol, ipratropium bromide and budesonide nebs. She tells you she can't breathe and is obviously short of breath.

---

4. You are called urgently to see Mr Gumble (52), a long-term alcoholic, has just vomited copious quantities of bright red blood for the 5th time in 20 minutes. The nurse tells you he feels cold, has a heart rate of 140 and a BP 90 / 50.

---

5. A 24-year old with Down's syndrome was admitted with a chest infection and commenced on co-amoxiclav. You are called because his temperature is now 39.1°c, and the nurses think you should take blood cultures. He's drowsy and you think he doesn't seem too well.

6. Mary Ryan is a 68-year old who is day 2 following aorto-femoral bypass and gives an 8-hour history of shortness of breath and central chest heaviness. She has no other past medical history, but appears very short of breath, and is sweating profusely.

7. Mr Smith is a 74-year old who was admitted 10 days ago with acute exacerbation of his COPD. He responded well to treatment with oxygen, regular salbutamol and ipratropium bromide nebulisers, co-amoxiclav and prednisolone and is waiting for a bed in a nursing home. You are asked to prescribe something to settle him down, as he appears very agitated and short of breath tonight.

Scenarios (with answers)

1.   You are called to see a 38-year old patient who has been admitted following an overdose of diazepam and alcohol. His GCS was 11 on admission, but is now 8. The nurses are concerned that he is making loud snoring noises and his oxygen saturations are 88% on room air.

*Assess ABCs. In this case – stop at A. His deteriorating conscious level means his **airway is compromised**. Management – **airway opening manoeuvres, Guedel or nasopharyngeal airway, high-flow oxygen. Roll the patient on their side to reduce risk of aspiration.** Call for help. Finish your ABCD assessment, addressing any other problems you find, obtain IV access and consider flumazenil to reverse the benzodiazepines. Arterial Blood Gas – hypoventilation will make CO_2 rise before O_2 falls, so he may already have a respiratory acidosis. Chest X-ray – has he already aspirated? Don't forget to finish your assessment after ABCD - secondary survey.*

2.   You are asked to admit a 45-year old asthmatic patient, who is complaining of chest tightness and breathlessness. She has been given a 5mg salbutamol nebuliser, which helped a little. Her SpO_2 is 95% but she is wheezy and unable to complete sentences due to breathlessness and has a respiratory rate of 32 / min.

Assess Airway – clear since she can complain!
*Breathing – Look, feel, listen and check SpO_2. Although SpO_2 maintained at present, she has life-threatening features of **acute severe asthma**.*
*Management - **High-flow oxygen.** Check PEFR if possible.*
*Nebulisers – **salbutamol 5mg continuously** depending on response, Ipratropium bromide 500 mcg as one-off.*
Assess circulation - look, feel, listen and monitor BP and ECG. Obtain IV access. These patients may be septic or grossly dehydrated and may require fluid resuscitation
IV Hydrocortisone 100-200mg or oral Prednisolone 40mg.
Check ABG, FBP, U+E, Mg, CRP, ECG, CXR.
IV antibiotics if evidence of infection.
* **Magnesium infusion 8mmol/30 mins unless rapid response to nebulisers. Consider Salbutamol or Aminophylline and in view of Life-threatening features:***

Refer to ICU unless rapid improvement. *See British Thoracic Society guidelines.*

3.   You are called to see Mrs Jones (73) in the fractures ward where she is day 1 following left hip hemiarthroplasty. Her current medications include furosemide, rampiril, and spironolactone tablets, and salbutamol, ipratropium bromide and budesonide nebs. She tells you she can't breathe and is obviously short of breath.

Assess ABCD
Tells you 'can't breathe'- so airway clear.
Breathing look, listen, feel and check SpO$_2$
From the history, this patient is on treatment for **heart failure** *and* **obstructive airways** *disease, giving two likely differential diagnoses already.* **Pulmonary embolus, pneumonia, atelectasis** *are other potential diagnoses.*
Remember there aren't many common causes of acute shortness of breath.
If she is unwell, treat according to clinical findings, otherwise you may be able to wait for the investigations
Don't forget to complete the assessment of C and D before a full secondary survey

4.   You are called urgently to see Mr Gumble (52), a long-term alcoholic, has just vomited copious quantities of bright red blood for the 5th time in 20 minutes. The nurse tells you he feels cold, has a heart rate of 140 and a BP 90 / 50.

Assess Airway and Breathing quickly
Circulation –Assess using the look/feel/listen/check BP and ECG. He has a history compatible with **hypovolaemic shock***. Management should consist of obtaining good IV access, commencing* **rapid fluid resuscitation***, and obtaining* **crossmatched blood** *urgently. As an alcoholic,* **varices** *are a likely diagnosis, so treat with a PPI, Terlipressin, restoration of normal coagulation and temperature, and refer urgently for endoscopy. Consider Sengstaken tube if there is a delay. Watch for decreased cerebral perfusion leading to decreased conscious level and airway compromise.*

3.   A 24-year old with Down's syndrome, was admitted with a chest infection and commenced on oral amoxicillin. You are called because his temp is now 39.1, blood pressure is low, and the nurses think you should take blood cultures. He's drowsy and you think he doesn't seem too well.

Assess ABCD
Airway – is he so drowsy that his airway is compromised? Give high flow oxygen.
Breathing – look/feel/listen/check SpO$_2$ and treat accordingly
Circulation – look/feel/listen/check BP and ECG

This patient is drowsy and pyrexial – likely diagnoses include meningitis, encephalitis, and severe sepsis originating from another source (eg pneumonia) leading to decreased cerebral perfusion. **Septic shock** *needs urgent and* **aggressive fluid resuscitation***, appropriate* **antibiotics***, and early referral to* **intensive care***.*

6.   Mary Ryan is a 68-year old who is day 2 following aorto-femoral bypass and gives an 2-hour history of shortness of breath and central chest heaviness. She has no other past medical history, but appears very short of breath, and is sweating profusely.

ABCD
Oxygen
IV access
ECG

*The likely diagnosis is **myocardial ischaemia and pulmonary oedema** but others (eg pulmonary embolus, tachyarrhythmia leading to myocardial ischaemia) should be considered*
Treatment may include:
Nitrates
Morphine
Aspirin
Furosemide
Discussion should take place between cardiologist and surgeon about anticoagulation if needed
Thrombolysis is contraindicated so primary PCI would be the treatment of choice for STEMI as well as NSTEMI

7.   Mr Smith is a 74-year old who was admitted 10 days ago with acute exacerbation of his COPD. He responded well to treatment with oxygen, regular salbutamol and Ipratropium bromide nebulisers, co-amoxiclav and prednisolone and is waiting for a bed in a nursing home. You are asked to prescribe something to settle him down, as he appears very agitated and short of breath tonight.

Go to see the patient
Assess ABCD
Agitation may well be a manifestation of hypoxia. Sedation will cause deterioration
*This patient will most likely need **oxygen** and treatment of COPD with nebulisers, steroids, and antibiotics if there is evidence of infection with consideration of early ventilatory support if unresponsive to medical therapy.*

PSYCHIATRY

General Psychiatric History and Mental State Assessment

		Not done	Adequate	Good
1	Introduces him/herself, his/her role and the purpose of the consultation	0	1	2
2	Confirms the patient's name, age, marital status, religion and occupation	0	1	2
3	Assesses patient's reason for presentation	0	1	2
4	Explores the Presenting Complaint and History of the Presenting complaint	0	1	2
5	Asks whether there is any family history of mental illness	0	1	2
6	Past psychiatric and past medical history	0	1	2
7	Drug history and allergies	0	1	2
8	Forensic history	0	1	2
9	Substance use history (alcohol and drugs)	0	1	2
10	Personal history to include: Birth and infancy Schooling and friendships Personal relationships Occupational history and relationships Current social circumstances	0	1	2
11	Premorbid personality	0	1	2
12	Assess the Mental State (including insight)	0	1	2
13	Assess their Suicide risk	0	1	2
14	Summarise back to patient	0	1	2
15	Does all the above appropriately and in an overtly empathic and non-judgemental manner	0		2

1. It is good practice to identify yourself, your and role and confirm the identity of the patient. Explain is simple terms the reason you are having the consultation.
2. These are all important factors which should be assessed early in the interview.
3. Are they there as a referral by another clinician. Have they attended due to a suggestion or influence from a relative or friend? Have the police or the courts or social services made it necessary for them attend? Have come seeking help? If they were referred, is this information provided in a referral letter.
4. You should use the patient's own words and explore the patient's priorities. Use open-ended questions. Explore especially;
   The nature of the problem
   The date of onset and speed of onset.
   Were there any precipitating factors, such as life events, illness etc?

The severity of this presentation and whether there has been any impact on work and relationships, as well as any physical effects, such as poor sleep, loss of weight or appetite and any psychosexual effects
Previous episodes similar to this, including treatments and outcomes, if the patient can remember.

It is after this section of the history the clinician can gauge and assess of the patient's level of insight. There is often some denial of the existence of a problem, but equally a patient may have a great deal of insight, which can at time be far more fear and distress provoking for the patient.

5. Here you should explore any pre-existing conditions, both medical and psychiatric among first and second degree relatives. It may be suitable to explore parental relationships here.

6. You should ask the patient to describe them self before they became unwell. You should focus on their mood and any particular character traits they mention. Ask the patient to describe their mood but also make your own assessment of their mood. Ask about previous medical conditions from childhood onwards.

7. Find out all the medications the patient is on (Prescribed, Herbal, Over the Counter). Do they have any allergies?

8. Ask whether they have ever encountered problems with law enforcement agencies (police, courts) and social services from childhood onwards. Has there been any violent behaviour?

9. Ask about level and pattern of alcohol intake (binge drinker, daytime drinker).

10. The personal history is a vast topic. A simple way to do this is to begin with birth and chilhood and then move through time until you reach the current problem. Thus you should explore
    Genetic factors such as any family history of mental illness.
    Parental history of alcohol or substance abuse.
    Pre-natal factors such as any maternal illness during pregnancy
    Any problems with the patient's actual delivery
    Any early childhood illnesses or problems
    Significant life events
        Schooling – bullying, friends, academic achievement
        Parental separation
        Further education
        Psychosexual development including any relationship and marital history
        Friendships
        Forensic history including any criminal records and previous episodes of violence or other acts of aggression.
        Employment; jobs held with reasons for changing or losing jobs. Assess their satisfaction with employment. Assess what effect that the illness will have on their job.

11. Ask when they felt completely well both physically and mentally.

12. Here the is a mnemonic that can help:

Always Be Sure To Assess Patient's Crazy Ideas

> **A**ppearance – are they appropriately dressed.
> **B**ehaviour - attitude to situation and clinician. Is it appropriate for the tone of the interview?
> **S**peech - rate, volume, quantity of information, disturbance in language or meaning
> **T**houghts - delusions, suicidal thoughts, continuity of ideas and pressure of ideas.
> **A**ffect - flattened, restricted, inappropriate
> **P**erception - hallucinations, depersonalisation, heightened or dulled perception
> **C**ognition - GCS, memory (immediate, recent and remote), orientation in time, place, person, concentration: count down from 100 in 7s.
> **I**nsight - individual's awareness of problem

There is also the Mini Mental State Exam, but this can take up to 10-15 minutes in itself. It is not suitable for making a diagnosis but can be used to indicate the presence of cognitive impairment.

13. See the separate chapter on suicide risk.

14. This is a useful tool, not only in emphasising that you are taking them and their problems seriously but also in making sure you have not missed or skipped over something they feel is important.

15. The better a rapport and level of trust you develop, the more the patient will open up and a good rapport has been shown to decrease the risk of relapse, as the patient will take more of what you have to say on board.

Psychiatric overview of symptoms

"**D**epressed **P**atients **S**eem **A**nxious, **S**o **C**laim **P**sychiatrists":
Depression and other mood disorders (major depression, bipolar disorder, dysthymia)
Personality disorders (primarily borderline personality disorder)
Substance abuse disorders
Anxiety disorders (panic disorder with agoraphobia, obssessive-compulsive disorder)
Somatization disorder, eating disorders (these two disorders are combined because both involve disorders of bodily perception)
Cognitive disorders (dementia, delirium)
Psychotic disorders (schizophrenia, delusional disorder and psychosis accompanying depression, substance abuse or dementia)

Depression History

		Not done	Adequate	Good
1	Makes an appropriate introduction	0	1	2
2	Explains the purpose of the interview	0	1	2
3	Clarifies the presenting complaint in terms of duration and any major life events that may have precipitated the illness	0	1	2
4	Explores their depressive symptoms including • Low mood, hopelessness • Poor sleep/early waking • Difficulty concentrating, loss of interest • Poor energy levels • Inability to have fun/enjoy things • Loss of appetite +/- weight • Bleak view of self/world/future • Deliberate self harm or suicidal intentions	0	1	2
5	Explores any past or family history of mental illness	0	1	2
6	Clarifies the past psychotic history, including medications and previous illnesses	0	1	2
7	Takes a detailed personal history, including job, alcohol, drugs and smoking	0	1	2
8	Uses appropriate non-verbal behaviour	0	1	2
9	Investigates any insight the patient may have	0	1	2
10	Summarises back to patient	0	1	2
11	Does all the above appropriately and in an overtly empathic manner	0	1	2

1. It is good practice to identify yourself, your and role and confirm the identity of the patient.

2. Explain is simple terms the reason you are having the consultation. Approach this sensitively, as a depressive patient may be very distressed and dealing with them with respect and empathy will help to build trust and rapport early in the consultation.

3. Use open-ended questions, but quickly narrow down on the diagnosis and look for supporting evidence. Find out the date of onset and was the onset slow or sudden? What precipitated the problem – work, loss/grieving and relationships are common causes. You should explore why and precisely how has the patient presented. Do they feel they are sad, depressed or were they motivated by something else, such as noticing they weren't sleeping well etc. Some patients may deny the existence of a problem and it may be necessary to obtain a collateral history.

4. These symptoms do not ALL have to occur for it to be depression, but the more that are the present, the higher your index of suspicion of depressive illness. You can always begin with open questions such as 'How have you been feeling in your mood or spirits recently?'
Be sure to be thorough in your exploration of their thoughts of suicide and self harm. This is done in greater detail in the Suicide Risk section.

5. A past or family history of a psychiatric disorder puts patients at higher risk of relapsing or developing their own mental health issue.

6. Have there been previous episodes? How were these treated and what were the outcomes. How were they generally before they became unwell in terms of mood, coping and life in general? Are they on any medications at all, both general and psychiatric?

7. The personal history should be as detailed as time will allow, starting as early as possible in the patients life. Talk about school, further education and jobs. Investigate any bullying or major life events in their past. Ask about whether they drink, smoke or use any illicit substance. You may at this point ask whether they have any forensic history.

8. Be as sensitive as possible in your non verbal behaviour. Attempt to appear open and non-judgmental.

9. Assess whether the patient recognises that there is something wrong and what they felt led up to it.

10. This is a useful tool, not only in emphasising that you are taking them and their problems seriously but also in making sure you have not missed or skipped over something they feel is important.

11. The better a rapport and level of trust you develop, the more the patient will open up and a good rapport has been shown to decrease the risk of relapse, as the patient will take more of what you have to say on board.

Schizophrenia Assessment

		Not done	Adequate	Good
1	Introduces self, and confirm identity of patient	0	1	2
2	Explains the purpose of the interview	0	1	2
3	Explores the presenting complaint in broad terms	0	1	2
4	Investigates the presence of any first rank symptoms of schizophrenia: a) Thought insertion b) Thought broadcasting c) Thought withdrawal d) Passivity phenomena e) Auditory hallucinations (3rd person/running commentary) f) Delusional perception	0	1	2
5	Investigates presence of other schizophrenic symptoms; a) Speech symptoms b) Affect c) Negative symptoms	0	1	2
6	Explores social history including drugs and alcohol	0	1	2
7	Investigates any thoughts of deliberate self harm or suicide	0	1	2
8	Explores any past or family history of mental illness	0	1	2
9	Investigates any precipitating life events	0	1	2
10	Uses appropriate non-verbal behaviour	0	1	2
11	Clarifies if the patient has any insight	0	1	2
12	Summarises back to patient	0	1	2
13	Does all the above appropriately and in an overtly empathic manner	0	1	2

1. It is very important in any psychiatry consultation to clarify you name and role and to be particularly sure you are talking to the correct patient. This is best done with name and date of birth.
2. It instantly develops a rapport to explain why you are there, especially with a schizophrenic patient who may be hyper-vigilant or paranoid
3. Patients with a higher IQ frequently have some insight, but this is never a definite. Explore fully the level of insight the patient has into their illness.
4. These symptoms must be explored fully:
   a. Do they feel thoughts are being placed in their head by an outside force?
   b. Do they feel as if their thoughts are being broadcast from their head to the external world where other people can hear them.
   c. A feeling that thoughts have been removed from their head, sometimes leaving the patient with a feeling that they are now lacking those thoughts and are somehow diminished by the process
   d. This can be a general feeling that thoughts, sensations and actions are under external control.
   e. These are perceptions in the absence of a stimulus. These tend to be auditory but may be visual or somatic in nature. They can be 2nd (a

voice talking to you) or 3rd (voices talking about you) or voices giving a running commentary or hearing your own thoughts echoed out aloud (thought echo).

    f. A delusion is a belief, amounting to a conviction that is held even when you present evidence to the contrary. They cannot be explained by culture, personality etc. The first rank type most commonly seen here might be an abnormal significance given to a normal event; 'the postman arrived and I realised I was the son of god'

5.

    a. Frequent derailment or incoherence; There may be interruptions to the flow of thought (thought blocking), loss of normal thought structure (knight's move thinking/word salad) and even neologisms (word, term, or phrase that the patient invents)

    b. The affect is the external representation of a person's mood, and a schizophrenic may be flattened, incongruous or just plain odd!

    c. These are so-named because they are the loss or absence of normal traits or abilities, and include blunted affect and emotions, poverty of speech, a lack of motivation and an inability to enjoy things (alogia, avolition and anhedonia respectively)

6. Alcohol and substance misuse has been associated with schizophrenia and schizophrenia like symptoms and it has also been noted that schizophrenics who are violent frequently are also substance abusers. Social drift is also a common finding in patients suffering from schizophrenia.

7. One must rule out the possibility that the patient is having thoughts of DSH. Many patients with insight become depressed and it is always possible that their auditory hallucinations may be suggesting DSH. Also psychotic depression is a differential diagnosis with a patient like this and again are at a high risk of DSH. A schizophrenic will tend to live 10 years less than an average person on the street due to the DSH rates and other health implications.

8. A past or family history of psychiatric illness, especially schizophrenia increases the risk significantly that this may be a schizophrenic illness.

9. There is an association found in schizophrenia with primary birth complications including infection in utero ett.

10. This can be done in a very open manner, "Do you think you might be unwell?" or perhaps, if you feel it is appropriate, "why do you think you are in hospital" or a similar phrase.

11, 12, 13. Obtaining a history of schizophrenia is a very sensitive matter. Time should be taken to make sure no undue distress is caused to the patient. The rapport is vital and regular pauses should be made for the patient to have thinking time, after which you may summarise back if you feel it is appropriate.

Deliberate Self Harm and Suicide Assessment

		Not done	Adequate	Good
1	Introduces self and role	0	1	2
2	Explains the purpose of the interview	0	1	2
3	Establish events leading up to attempt	0	1	2
4	Establishes method and uses *Abridged Pierce Suicide Intent Scale*[1] a) Isolation b) Timing c) Precautions against rescue d) Acting to gain help e) Final acts in anticipation f) Suicide note g) Lethality h) Stated intent i) Premeditation j) Reaction to act k) Predictable Outcome l) Death without medical treatment	0	1	2
5	Establish previous or family history of self harm or psychiatric illness	0	1	2
6	Explore alcohol, cigarette and drug usage	0	1	2
7	Explore personality and mood; Premorbid and current	0	1	2
8	Use of appropriate non-verbal and verbal style	0	1	2
9	Makes explicit empathic statements	0	1	2
10	May have to demonstrate an understanding of the basic tenants of sectioning a patient	0	1	2
11	Does the above in a organised and systematic fashion	0	1	2

1. Clarify your name and your role, as well as confirming the identity of the patient
2. This is a sensitive topic, but is best dealt with in a straightforward, but empathic, way. Having explored why they feel they are in hospital you should move on to the reason for your consultation. If the doctor shows no embarrassment then the patient is less likely to, "Is ok if we talk about your thoughts about hurting yourself" or "I'm here to talk about the overdose you took last night, I know this is difficult but is that ok?"
3. You have to explore their reason for their suicidal thoughts or attempt. Have there been any recent negative events such as a divorce/break-up, redundancy, diagnosis of serious illness or loss of a relative? Do they live alone? Are they suffering chronic pain? Are they having any financial difficulties and finally have they been or are they soon to be imprisoned?
4. These should be explored in depth. The answers go up in terms of risk, so for example, "someone present" is a low risk whereas "no one nearby" is a high risk. After clarifying the basic method of attempt, i.e. cutting, hanging, overdose etc, use the following table to assess their risk.

1	Isolation	Someone present, Someone nearby or on telephone, No-one nearby
2	Timing	Timed so intervention likely, probable intervention unlikely, intervention highly unlikely
3	Precautions against rescue	None, Passive (e.g. alone in room, door unlocked), Active precautions
4	Acting to gain help	Notifies helper of attempt, Contacts helper, doesn't tell, No contact with helper
5	Final acts in anticipation	None, Partial preparation, Definite plans (e.g. will, insurance, gifts)
6	Suicide note	None, Note torn up, Presence of note
7	Lethality	Thought would not kill, Unsure if lethal action, Believed would kill
8	Stated intent	Did not want to die, Unsure, Wanted to die
9	Premeditation	Impulsive, Considered less than 1 hour, Considered less than 1 day, Considered more than 1 day
10	Reaction to act	Glad recovered, Uncertain, Sorry he/she failed
11	Predictable outcome	Survival certain, Death unlikely, Death likely or certain
12	Death without medical treatment	No, Uncertain, Yes

5. Any past history or family history of either psychiatric illness or actual deliberate self harm increases the suicide risk overall
6. Substance misuse is associated with an increased suicide risk, and this includes alcoholism
7. Explore fully their condition up to either their attempt or if no attempt has been made, up to their suicidal ideas began. This also gives a good indication of their current mood and the likelihood they will either go ahead with their attempt or repeat the act. Use simple questions such as;

- Do you derive any pleasure from your life?
- How do you feel about facing each day?
- Do you see any point in life?
- Do you ever feel that you can't face tomorrow?
- Do you know why you feel this way?
- Have you done anything about it other than this attempt?
- Is there anyone who you can ask for help?

If the consultation is post-suicide attempt, you should always ask a variation on "Are you going to try to end your life again?"

8. The formation of a good relationship, with an empathic and reassuring manner and questioning style will make for a much easier consultation and will reduced patient anxiety.
9. In scenarios such as this, you have to be overt in showing that you appreciate the way someone must be feeling to resort to ending their life.
10. You may be asked what you feel is best for this patient in which case you should understand the basics of the Mental Health Act in terms of sectioning patients. It is recommended you understand the indications for each of these and who is required to acquire such a section but also that a section is not always needed and that you can treat a patient under Common Law;

Section 2: Admission for assessment
Section 3: Admission for treatment (up to 6 months)
Section 4: Emergency treatment (for up to 72 hours)
Section 5(2): Detention of a patient already in hospital (up to 72 hours)
Section 5(4): Nurses' holding-powers (for up to 6 hours)
Section 20(4): Renewal of compulsory detention in hospital
Section 136 (for up to 72 hours) by Police

11. This consultation is a challenging one and having an organised approach will make it less difficult for you and the patient!

EYES
AND
FUNDOSCOPY

Examination of the Eyes

		Not Attempted	Attempted inadequate	Attempted adequate
1.	Introduces self, explains role and obtains consent	0	1	2
2.	Asks about presenting complaint and history of presenting complaint and brief past medical history.	0	1	2
3.	Wears gloves or washes hands with an antiseptic lotion.	0	1	2
4	Places patient in good light or has torch for examination	0	1	2
5.	Inspects the eyebrows, eyelids, eyelashes and the orbital area	0	1	2
6.	Palpates the eyelids for nodules (eyes closed)	0	1	2
7	Palpates the lacrimal gland in the superior temporal orbital rim (both eyes)	0	1	2
8.	Pulls down the lower eyelid gently and inspects the conjunctivae and sclerae (both eyes). Pulls the upper eyelid upwards and inspects the sclerae (both eyes).	0	1	2
9.	Separates eyelids gently with index finger and thumb (left hand for right eye and vice versa) and inspects the cornea and anterior chamber. Uses torch judiciously. (Both eyes). Checks papillary size, shape and responses to light and accommodation. Checks corneal sensitivity.	0	1	2
10.	Inspects both eyes for squint, muscle balance and nystagmus. Performs cover/uncover test.	0	1	2
11.	Inspects range of eye movements in a systematic fashion	0	1	2
12.	Performs fundoscopy	0	1	2
13.	Measures visual acuity for near vision, distant	0	1	2

	vision, peripheral vision and colour vision.			
14.	Thanks patients, removes gloves and washes hands.	0	1	2

1. It is polite to introduce yourself, explain why you are there and get verbal consent for the examination.
2. Ask what the presenting complaint is and ask for a brief history of presenting complaint. Ask regarding hypertension or diabetes and any previous conditions affecting the eyes or eyesight.
3. It is best to wear gloves but some feel it reduces the sensitivity of the fingers. An alternative is to wash your hands and rub with an antiseptic lotion.
4. For external eye examination good ambient light is essential. For examination of the cornea, anterior chamber and pupils a torch is essential.
5. Inspect the eyebrows for hair texture and symmetry. Inspect eyelashes for extensions and cosmetic use, ectropion and entropion (eversion or inversion). Inspect eyelids for oedema, droop (ptosis), puffiness, fasciculations, flakiness, redness and swelling (blepharitis). Look at the periorbital skin for rashes, eczema or lesions. Basal Cell Carcinomas often arise below the medial canthus. Ask patient to open and close eyelids completely and observe their movement.
6. Palpate the eyelids for nodules (eyelash follicultis=stye) or chalazion (inflamed meibomian gland).
7. The lacrimal gland lies above the lateral canthus but the lacrimal apparatus and duct opening is at the medial canthus. If the lacrimal duct is blocked, the eye will become dry and sore and the lacrimal gland may become palpable.
8. Look for pallor (anaemia), inflammation (conjunctivitis), pterygium (encroachment of the conjunctiva onto the cornea). Blue scleare may be associated with Osteogenesis imperfecta or Marfan's or Ehlers Danlos syndrome and yellow sclerae is a sign of obstructive jaundice.
9. Look at the eye with a torch. The cornea should be clear (no opacities) and should not have any blood vessels over it. Corneal arcus is the presence of lipid deposits in the periphery of the cornea and may be associated with hyperlipidaemia. Look at the iris for colour, pupillary shape, contour, uniformity and symmetry. Look at the anterior chamber (space between the cornea and iris) for dependant blood (hyphaema). Miosis is pupillary constriction (opiates, anti-glaucoma drugs), mydriasis is pupillary dilatation (mydriatic eye drops, coma, brain injury) and anisocoria is unequal papillary size. The pupillary reflex is direct and consensual (shining a light on the right pupil will constrict both pupils). The corneal reflex is a blink in response to touching with a wisp of sterile cotton wool.
10. Ask the patient to look straight ahead and shine a light at the bridge of the nose, look at the reflection of light in both corneas, it should be at the same level both horizontally and vertically. Cover-uncover test looks at the presence of a squint. Ask the patient to focus on a small object, cover one eye and after a few seconds, uncover. If the uncovered eye moves to see the object, a squint should be suspected.
11. Ask the patient to look at your index finger and move it in the form of the letter 'H'. Each part of the movement checks a particular set of muscles. You should know the muscles supplied by the Abducens, Oculomotor and Trochlear nerves and the movements of the eyeball caused by these muscles. A helpful link: http://en.wikipedia.org/wiki/Eye_movements
12. See separate section on fundoscopy.

13. Use standard charts for testing visual acuity (Snellen's) and colour vision (Ishihara charts). Peripheral vision is tested by the 'confrontation' test: Sit or stand at eye level with the subject. Ask them to stare at your Right eye with their left eye (and vice versa). Extend your arm, wiggle your finger and ask them to tell you when the can see the movements. Test Nasal, Temporal, Superior and Inferior fields in turn.

14. Always wash your hands after every examination.

FUNDOSCOPY

		Not done	Adequate	Good
1	Introduces self, gains consent and confirms identity of patient. Describes procedure to patient.	0	1	2
2	Prepares ophthalmoscope correctly	0	1	2
3	Darkens room, has patient look up at a specific point on the wall	0	1	2
4	To examine R eye, holds ophthalmoscope in R hand, and looks with R eye; vice versa for left eye. Checks focusing wheel is at zero.	0	1	2
5	Keeps index finger on focusing wheel and keeps other hand on patient's fore head or shoulder	0	1	2
6	Tries to keep both of his/her eyes open. Starts one foot away from the patient.	0	1	2
7	Assess the red reflex; note uniformity of colour, shadows	0	1	2
8	Moves in towards eye at 15 degrees laterally until about 2 inches from eye	0	1	2
9	Turns focusing wheel to bring retina into focus	0	1	2
10	Uses minus lenses if the patient is myopic, plus lenses if hyperopic	0	1	2
11	Examines the optic disc	0	1	2
12	Examine the retinal vessels	0	1	2
13	Examines the retinal background	0	1	2
14	Examines the macula	0	1	2
15	Describes findings in an organised fashion	0	1	2
16	Thanks patient and washes hands	0	1	2

1. This is the standard procedure before any examination. Explain you will be shining a bright light into their eyes, they should not look at this light unless told to and that you will be getting very close to their face.

2. Confirm it has enough battery power to supply sufficient light. Small aperture of light for undilated pupil, large aperture for dilated pupil . Red-free filter – to visualize blood vessels and haemorrhages

3. This can be arbitrary so long as it is easily identifiable, e.g. light switch, book shelf etc.

4. This is the best way to get close enough to the patient. Fundoscopy is, by nature an intimate exam and this should be at the forefront of the candidate's thoughts. Some examiners will change the setting on the fundoscope between students.

5. The hand on the forehead both reassures the patient and keeps their head still, as they are likely to flinch as you get closer to their face.

6. This is a skill that develops with practice. You do not want to be stood on the other side of the room, there is no advantage to this.

7. At times opacities can be seen at this stage. Red reflex is absent in lens opacity (cataract), detached retina or artificial eye, an examiners favourite!).

8. This is so it does not appear that you are heading straight for the patient's eye, which is threatening for the patient but also is the best position for the later stages including identifying the optic disc. If you have approached 15° lateral, you should now be seeing the retina in the vicinity of the optic disc.

9. If able to see the optic disc, bring it in to sharp focus

10. Short sighted patient (myopic). Long sighted patient (hyperopic).

11. To find optic disc (nasal to centre of retina), follow a blood vessel as it widens. Note any margin distinction, colour, symmetry, haemorrhages, elevation, cup to disc ratio (normal < 0.5)

12. Follow vessels to the periphery, note arteriovenous crossings; arteries are lighter-coloured, thinner, and have a brighter reflex than veins

13. Note the colour (normal = red-orange), pigmentation, and lesions (flame-shaped, diffuse spotting, cotton wool spots)

14. To find the macula, move the light two disc diameters temporally, or ask patient to look directly into light; it should be avascular with a light reflex at fovea; may be darker in colour than rest of retina

15. Explain your findings in term of anatomy and quadrants, e.g the superior nasal quadrant or inferior temporal quadrant.

16. It is polite to thank the patient. Always wash your hands to reduce the risk of cross-infection.

EAR, NOSE
AND
THROAT

EXAMINATION OF THE EARS

		Not Attempted	Attempted inadequate	Attempted adequate
1.	Introduces self, explains role and gains consent	0	1	2
2.	Positions patient correctly and in good light	0	1	2
3.	Inspects the auricles and mastoid area	0	1	2
4	Asks patient if ears are tender and gently palpates the auricles and mastoid area			
5	Inspects the auditory canal with an otoscope	0	1	2
6.	Inspects the tympanic membrane	0	1	2
7.	Assesses hearing			
8	Performs Weber and Rinne tests with a tuning fork.	0	1	2
9	Thanks patient and washes hands			

1. It is important to introduce yourself, explain your role in their care and explain what you are about to do.
2. Sit the patient up on a revolving stool as this allows 360 degree access to their ears, head and neck. Either have a headlight on or use focused external light to illuminate the head and neck.
3. Inspect the pinna, external auditory meatus and mastoid area for size, shape, symmetry (compare both sides), landmarks, position and deformities or other abnormalities and skin lesions. Cauliflower ear is caused by trauma and necrosis of the cartilage of the pinna. Tophi are small whitish crystals of uric acid which may be associated with gout.
4. Palpate the pinna and mastoid area for tenderness, swelling and nodules.
5. Tilt the patient's head towards the opposite shoulder and gently pull the pinna upwards and backwards, this straightens the external auditory canal. Look for wax, colour, skin lesions, inflammation, discharge and foreign bodies. Wax should be odourless.
6. Look for landmarks (annulus is the ring around the tympanic membrane and umbo is the area in the centre of the tympanic membrane that is pulled in by the malleus), colour, contour, perforations and mobility.
7. Assess hearing by responses to instructions during the examination and response to whispered voice and finger rub.
8. Weber test: Strike a tuning fork (512 Hz) and place the stem of the fork on the top of the patient's skull - equal distance from the patient's ears, in the middle of the forehead - equal distance from the patient's ears or above the upper lip over the teeth. Ask the patient in which ear the sound is heard louder.
Rinne test: Place a vibrating tuning fork (512 Hz) initially on the mastoid process until sound is no longer heard, then move the fork immediately just outside the ear. Normally, the sound is audible at the ear.

It is polite to thank the patient. Always wash your hands to reduce the risk of cross-infection.

EXAMINATION OF THE NOSE AND SINUSES

		Not Attempted	Attempted inadequate	Attempted adequate
1.	Introduces self, explains role and gains consent	0	1	2
2.	Positions patient correctly and in good light	0	1	2
3.	Inspects the external nose	0	1	2
4	Asks patient if nose is tender and gently palpates the ridge and soft tissues of the nose			
5.	Looks for patency of the nares	0	1	2
6.	Inspects the nasal mucosa and nasal septum with nasal separator			
7	Inspects frontal and maxillary sinuses	0	1	2
8.	Palpates and percusses the frontal and maxillary sinuses	0	1	2
9	Thanks patient and washes hands	0	1	2

1. It is important to introduce yourself, explain your role in their care and explain what you are about to do.
2. Sit the patient up on a revolving stool as this allows 360 degree access to their nose, head and neck. Either have a headlight on or use focused external light to illuminate the head and neck.
3. Inspect for shape, size, colour, contour and look at the nares.
4. Palpate for tenderness, displacement of cartilage and bone and any masses.
5. Put your thumb or index finger on the tip of the nose and gently lift upwards to look closely at the nares and assess their patency.
6. Look at the colour of the mucosa, alignment of the septum, discharge, swelling of the turbinates, perforation or polyps. Unilateral watery discharge after trauma indicates fracture of the cribriform plate. Bilateral discharge is due to rhinitis. Bloodstained discharge is due to trauma or tumours.
7. Look for redness or swelling.
8. Look for swelling and tenderness.
9. It is polite to thank the patient. Always wash your hands to reduce the risk of cross-infection.

EXAMINATION OF THE MOUTH

		Not Attempted	Attempted inadequate	Attempted adequate
1.	Introduces self, explains role and gains consent	0	1	2
2.	Positions patient correctly and in good light	0	1	2
3.	Dons gloves and inspects and gently palpates the lips with the index finger	0	1	2
4	Inspects and gently palpates the gums			
5.	Inspects the teeth	0	1	2
6.	Inspects tongue and oral mucosa			
7	Checks tongue movements	0	1	2
8.	Palpates the tongue	0	1	2
9.	Inspects the soft and hard palate and the uvula			
10.	Inspects the tonsils and posterior wall of the pharynx			
11.	Thanks patient, removes gloves and washes hands.			

1. It is important to introduce yourself, explain your role in their care and explain what you are about to do.

2. Sit the patient up on a revolving stool as this allows 360 degree access to their nose, head and neck. Either have a headlight on or use focused external light to illuminate the head and neck.

3. Look at shape, colour, contour and oedema. Cheilitis is dry cracked lips at the angles of the mouth. Cheilosis is deep fissures at the angles of the mouth (riboflavin deficiency). Pale lips indicate anaemia. Cherry red lips indicate acidosis or carbon monoxide poisoning. Blue lips indicate peripheral cyanosis. Circumoral pigmentation is a feature of the Peutz-Jeughers syndrome (intestinal polyps). Nicotine stained lips and moustache indicate prolonged heavy smoking.

4&5. Look for tenderness, colour and surface bleeding of the gums and caries, missing teeth and occlusion. You will need a mirrored speculum for this.

6. Look at the colour of the mucosa, symmetry and contour of the tongue, furring or discoloration. Geographical tongue is a patchy discolouration of the tongue caused by a variety of reasons including infections and allergies. Furring of the tongue may indicate gastrointestinal infection. Whitish plaques with inflamed edges indicate a fungal infection and may be seen in patients who have been on prolonged courses of antibiotics. Leukoplakia of the tongue or oral mucosa is the presence of a discrete white patch. Squamous cancers of the tongue or oral mucosa may present as an ulcer with rolled pearly edges.

7. Note any atrophy or fasciculations of the tongue while it is resting on the floor of the mouth. Ask the patient to stick their tongue straight out and note whether it curves to one side or the other. Ask the patient to move their tongue from side to side and push it forcefully against the inside of each cheek. Fasciculations and atrophy are signs of lower motor neuron lesions. Unilateral tongue weakness causes the tongue to deviate toward the weak side. Tongue weakness can result from lesions of the tongue muscles, the neuromuscular junction, the lower motor neurons of the

hypoglossal nerve, or the upper motor neurons originating in the motor cortex. Lesions of the motor cortex cause contralateral tongue weakness.

8. Palpate gently so not to elicit the gag reflex.

9&10. A good technique is to wrap the tip of the tongue in a piece of gauze and gently pull it out of the mouth, this gives a good view of the tonsils and pharynx.

11. It is polite to thank the patient. Always wash your hands to reduce the risk of cross-infection.

GYNAECOLOGY AND OBSTETRICS

General gynaecological history

		Not Attempted	Attempted inadequate	Attempted adequate
1.	Introduces self to patient, explains role and gains consent	0	1	2
2.	Asks patients name age and occupation	0	1	2
3.	Asks what the presenting complaint is.	0	1	2
4.	Ask about age of onset of menarche	0	1	2
5.	Asks whether the patient has regular periods, the interval between periods and cycle duration	0	1	2
6.	Asks whether there has been any changes to her cycle	0	1	2
7.	Asks LMP and whether there is a chance she could be pregnant	0	1	2
8.	Asks about dysmenorrhoea	0	1	2
9.	Asks about mennorrhagia	0	1	2
10.	Asks about intermenstrual bleeding	0	1	2
11.	Asks if patient is sexually active (multiple partners)	0	1	2
12.	Asks about dysparenuria	0	1	2
13.	Asks about post coital bleeding	0	1	2
14.	Asks about contraception	0	1	2
15.	Asks about vaginal discharge	0	1	2
16.	Asks about whether she is ever incontinent of urine	0	1	2
17.	Asks about history of prolapse (sensation of something coming down)	0	1	2
18.	Ask history of operations on abdomen or pelvis	0	1	2
19.	Asks whether she has any children and whether she wishes to in the future	0	1	2
20.	Asks about previous pregnancies and outcomes			
21.	Asks whether she's ever had screening for, or a diagnosis of STI	0	1	2
22.	Asks date of last smear and if she's ever had an	0	1	2

	abnormal smear			
23.	Ask if her or any of her family have ever had breast cancer, gynaecological cancers, difficulty conceiving or thyroid problems			
24.	Asks about past / current medication and allergies			
25.	Asks about smoking, alcohol and drug abuse			
26.	Asks about home circumstances			

1) It is polite to introduce yourself, explain why you are there and get verbal consent from the patient.

2) Asking the patient's name allows you to identify the patient
Age can affect the likely diagnosis e.g. the commonest cause of mennorrhagia in a young girl is anovulatory cycles, or in a perimenopausal woman there is a risk of endometrial carcinoma (15% risk in postmenopausal bleeding). The date of birth should be recorded to identify the patient.

3) Asking why the patient has come to hospital/clinic/ G.P allows you to conduct a patient centred interview, addressing their problems before completing your questions.

4) Early menarche (onset of menstruation) and overall length of menstruation is related to an increased risk of endometrial cancer

5) A normal cycle is measured from the 1st day of the menstrual period to the onset of the next menstrual period. It can vary from 22-35 days in length and bleeding should last less than 7 days. This is written as k= number of days bleeding / days in the cycle (e.g. if a women bleeds for 5 days every 28 days k= 5/28). Oligomennorrhoea is infrequent periods occurring less than every 35 days. Amenorrhoea is absence of periods in a woman of reproductive age and is either primary (never started e.g. Turners syndrome, vaginal obstruction, Prader-Willi etc) or secondary (suddenly ceased). Secondary amenorrhoea can be due to normal physiological events such as pregnancy, menopause or due to pathology affecting the hypothalamus (weight loss, excessive exercise, stress), pituitary (pituitary tumours), ovaries (polycystic ovaries), uterus (Asherman's syndrome) or thyroid dysfunction.

6) A recent change in cycle could be due to physical upset, psychological upset, pregnancy, pelvic inflammatory disease or any of the causes of secondary amenorrhoea.

7) It's important to check she is not pregnant. The date of her last menstrual period may be relevant for management options.

8) Dysmenorrhoea (painful periods) is a common problem. It's important to establish the timing of this. It is important to elicit whether this is associated with her cycle; Does it come on with her period or does she get it days before her period? The latter is associated with PID, endometriosis (pathological causes of painful periods) and fibroids (non-cyclical pain). Does the pain limit activities or require medication? This gives a good indication of severity of the pain. The use of analgesics is common and should be documented.

9) Ask about menorrhagia (heavy periods) and flooding which can be associated with fibroids, endometriosis, clotting disorders, carcinoma, PID etc. Clarify this by asking how many tampons and/or pads she uses per day. Getting out of bed at night to change pads is a good indicator of menorrhagia.

10) Intermenstrual bleeding can be caused by lesions of the vulva (ulcers, cancer), vagina (local trauma, atrophic vaginitis), cervix (polyps, carcinoma or an ectropion), lesions of the uterine body (endometriosis, fibroids, polyps, carcinoma) or by sexually transmitted diseases such as Chlamydia.

11) Sexually active females with multiple partners may become pregnant, can be at risk of STD's and have increased risk of CIN and cervical cancer.

12) Ask about deep and superficial dyspareunia (painful sexual intercourse). Causes include episiotomy, recurrent infection, herpes zoster, gland pathology, cystitis, dryness (especially during menopause), endometriosis, retroverted uterus and psychological causes.

13) Ask about bleeding after sex. This can be due to lesions or the cervix or from sexually transmitted diseases e.g. Chlamydia. Atrophic vaginitis can cause post-coital bleeding.

14) It's important to check the patient is using adequate contraception, both in terms of protection against pregnancy and STI's. Discuss the options with her if she wishes.

15) See vaginal discharge history.

16) See point 7 on general urological history. Urine leakage is common in women after childbirth and with infections. Pelvic floor exercises can help reduce the likelihood of this. Ascertain whether she has stress or urge incontinence.

17) Uterovaginal prolapse is rare before the menopause (oestrogen is protective). It can cause discomfort, discharge, bleeding and urinary symptoms.

18) Abdominal/pelvic surgery can lead to adhesions, which in turn can cause pain, infection and fertility issues. If they have had any such operations, these should be explored fully.

19) It's important to establish this as it may effect the differential diagnosis and the management options e.g. a hysterectomy for menorrhagia could only be considered if the patient had completed her family.

20) Ask parity (live births, stillbirths, miscarriages, abortions, and ectopics). See obstetric history.

21) STD's can have complications if left untreated e.g. untreated Chlamydia can lead to PID and possibly infertility.

22) History of an abnormal smear may give clues as to the underlying cause of any current complaints. This is a good opportunity to emphasise the importance of regular smears.

23) A patient treated with tamoxifen for breast cancer is at increased risk of endometrial cancer. Adenocarcinoma of the uterus can metastasise. Endometriosis and polycystic ovaries are occasionally discovered during investigations for infertility. Both hyper- and hypothyroidism can lead to disturbances of the menstrual cycle.

24) Its important to find out if the patient is taking HRT (hormone replacement therapy) or OCP(oral contraceptive pills) or other hormonal contraception. Depo-provera can cause irregular cycles and delayed fertility after discontinuation of treatment.

25) Smoking is a risk factor for cervical cancer and complications in pregnancy. "Risk taking behaviour" is also associated with higher risks of sexually transmitted diseases.

26) Many gynaecological conditions have detrimental effects on quality of life and on relationships. This should be considered in any management plan.

OBSTETRIC HISTORY

		Not Attempted	Attempted inadequate	Attempted adequate
1.	Introduces self to patient and obtains consent	0	1	2
2.	Asks patient's name, age, and occupation.	0	1	2
3.	Establishes reason for visit	0	1	2
4.	Asks: When was the pregnancy confirmed? Gestation at booking? Has she had a scan? If so when was the last scan?	0	1	2
5.	Asks dates of last menstrual period	0	1	2
6.	Ask about previous contraception – when last used? Has she been on OCP in last 6 months)	0	1	2
7.	Asks length of menstrual cycle and was it regular?	0	1	2
8.	Asks Gravity / Parity	0	1	2
9.	Is it a planned pregnancy? Was it spontaneous or assisted?	0	1	2
10.	Any difficulties conceiving?	0	1	2
11.	How do you and your partner feel about the pregnancy?	0	1	2
12.	Asks if the woman and her partner are related to each other? Asks paternal age.	0	1	2
13.	Asks about symptoms of early pregnancy	0	1	2
14.	Asks about investigations during this pregnancy	0	1	2
15.	Asks about complications with this or previous pregnancies	0	1	2
16.	Establishes past obstetrics history	0	1	2
17.	Establishes past gynaecological history	0	1	2
18.	Asks when last smear was done	0	1	2
19.	Past Medical History and review of systems	0	1	2
20.	Drug History, Folic acid intake and allergies	0	1	2
21.	Asks about family history	0	1	2

22.	Asks social history and smoking	0	1	2
23.	Asks the patient if there is anything else you ought to know?	0	1	2
24.	Demonstrates good communication throughout	0	1	2
25.	Thanks the patient	0	1	2

1) It is both polite and rapport building to greet a patient so the patient knows who you are and what your role is. Obtain verbal consent to take a history from them.

2) The age of the patient is very important in obstetrics. Women over 35 and below the age of 17 are at higher risk of medical complications during their pregnancy. Congenital abnormalities (e.g. Downs syndrome) are more common with advancing maternal age. The occupation of the patient can give an idea of the background of the patient and there may be risks associated with certain paternal occupations (e.g. janitors, mechanics and metalworkers)

3) It's important to know why the patient is here and their expectations of the consultation.

4) This will establish whether the pregnancy has been confirmed by a doctor.

5) Last menstrual period (LMP) allows you to work out EDD (Expected Date of Delivery) and gestation allowing you to plan the woman's antenatal care. A full term pregnancy lasts 280 days from the first day of the LMP. This assumes regular periods lasting 28 days.

6) Using the oral contraceptive pill (OCP) within 6 months before becoming pregnant can mask anovulatory cycles in predisposed women. Recent contraceptive use is important because i) recent OCP may render LMP as an assessment of gestation unreliable; ii) Patient may still have an intrauterine contraceptive device (IUCD) still in-situ; iii) indicates a failure of her contraceptive method in preventing her pregnancy.

7) Written as K = x/y (e.g If bleed for 4 days every 28 days k= 4/28).

8) Gravity describes the total number of pregnancies a woman has had, regardless as to whether they were carried to term. This is only used if the patient is currently pregnant. Parity refers to the number of deliveries > 24 weeks (live births and stillbirths). A suffix after the initial number describes the number of pregnancies < 24 weeks (miscarriages/ terminations of pregnancies and ectopics). For example a woman with 2 children and one previous miscarriage at 12 weeks, is classified as Para 2 + 1. If she was to fall pregnant again she would be classed as gravida 4 (para 2 + 1). A women who has delivered no live or potentially live babies is nulliparous,

9) Assisted conceptions carry greater risk of multiple births, miscarriages, ectopic pregnancies, as well as being associated with an increase in perinatal mortality and morbidity.

10) Ask if they've ever had any difficulty conceiving?

11) It is important to assess how the woman and her partner feel about the pregnancy and whether they have any worries or concerns.

12) Consanguineous marriages are more common in certain ethnic groups. They have a higher risk of genetic disorders and of perinatal mortality. Increasing paternal age can also increase the risk of congenital disorders.

13) Amenorrhoea, breast enlargement / morning sickness (hyperemesis gravidarum is an extreme form). Also urinary symptoms e.g. increased frequency. Food 'cravings'.

14) Has she had her blood sugar or blood pressure tested? Any blood tests, ultrasound scans or screening/diagnostic tests during this pregnancy.

15) Any bleeding, pain, hypertension, proteinuria, diabetes, anaemia, or urinary infection. Has anyone expressed any concerns about fetal growth or admissions to hospital during the pregnancy?

16) Ask the year, mode of delivery and the gestation. If there was an instrumental delivery or a caesarean section, what was the reason? Ask about any complications during the previous pregnancy. Ask the birth weight of the child and whether any resuscitation was needed for the child or any special care baby unit (SCBU) admissions?

17) Establish a past gynaecological history in brief: Ask about intermenstrual bleeding, post-coital bleeding, dysmenorrhoea, menorrhagia, previous history of any sexually transmitted disease or vaginal discharge.

18) Date of last smear. Check if one needs to be arranged for after the birth. Ask if they've ever had an abnormal smear.

19) Past Medical History and systematic review – ever been in hospital / had any operations? Ever had a blood transfusion (if so when)? Ask about rubella vaccination? Women with previous uterine surgery may require a caesarean section. Do a full system review including cardiac, respiratory, abdominal and neurological symptoms. Patients with serious medical conditions (especially epilepsy, diabetes and thyroid disorders) are more likely to encounter problems during their pregnancy and usually need input from the appropriate specialist.

20) Is the patient on any prescription or over the counter tablets, inhalers or injections? Have they taken pre-conceptual folic acid (it protects against some congenital abnormalities) and if so- for how long have they taken the supplement? Specifically ask about drugs taken after the last menstrual period (LMP). Don't forget to ask about allergies – specifically penicillin (either penicillin or cefuroxime and metronidazole is sometimes routinely given if the woman has a persistent pyrexia (>38^{0}C during labour) and latex. Any drugs that are contraindicated in pregnancy should be changed.

21) Ask about family history of multiple pregnancies, diabetes, hypertension, pre-eclampsia, thrombophilia, congenital diseases or inherited disorders.

22) Ask about smoking, alcohol, drug use and whether the patient is married or single. Asking "who's at home with you" is a nice way to initiate this. Find out the occupation of partner and whether they live in a house they own house or rented accommodation? Drug abuse is associated with preterm labour, increased perinatal mortality and drug dependence in the neonate. Smoking reduces fertility, increases the risk or miscarriage, placental abruption, perinatal death,and intra uterine growth restriction. Asking if the patient is married or in a long term relationship will give an indication of the level of social support available in the home. The Royal College of Obstetricians and Gynecologists recommends that the issue of domestic violence should be carefully explored as part of the full antenatal booking visit.

23) Open questions give the patient a chance to disclose any information they feel to be important and to express any concerns they may have.

24) Uses appropriate questioning, avoids jargon and summarises back to patient.

Bimanual and Smear

		Not Attempted	Attempted inadequate	Attempted adequate
1.	Introduces self, explains procedure and gains verbal consent	0	1	2
2.	Requests a chaperone	0	1	2
3.	Ensures patient has an empty bladder	0	1	2
4.	Assembles equipment, washes hands and wears gloves	0	1	2
5.	Adequately exposes patient while maintaining her dignity	0	1	2
6.	Correctly positions patient	0	1	2
7.	Inspects vulva	0	1	2
8.	Reassures the patient at this stage if normal	0	1	2
9.	Prepares speculum ensuring it's warm and lubricated	0	1	2
10.	Parts the labia with the non dominant hand	0	1	2
11.	WARNS the patient you will begin inserting the speculum	0	1	2
12.	Inserts the speculum using the correct technique	0	1	2
13.	Visualises the cervix and fixes the speculum	0	1	2
14.	Observes the cervix and vaginal walls for lesions and discharge	0	1	2
15.	Obtains specimens for culture and cytology	0	1	2
16.	Withdraws the speculum and disposes of in a clinical waste bin	0	1	2
17.	Proceeds to bimanual examination after explaining what he/she is going to do next	0	1	2
18.	Lubricates fingers	0	1	2

19.	Parts the labia and inserts lubricated index and middle fingers	0	1	2
20.	Examines the cervix and checks for cervical excitation	0	1	2
21.	Palpates the uterus and adnexal structures	0	1	2
22.	Allows the patient to dress, maintains patient dignity, thanks the patient and washes hands	0	1	2
23.	Demonstrates good technique and a good standard of communication	0	1	2

1. It's important to introduce yourself (give your full name and role). Explain that you would like to examine them internally and take some cells from the cervix. Explain each step to the patient before you do it.

2. Asking for a chaperone protects you as a doctor from any possible accusations and is a must for both males and females. This can also reassure the patient.

3. The speculum can put pressure on the bladder so ensure the patient has gone to the toilet before you start your examination.

4. Check instruments. You will need; smear fix, cervix brush and the correct sized speculum.

5. Adequately expose the patient by asking them to undress below the waist including their underwear. Maintain the patient's dignity by covering them with a blanket when are not being examined.

6. Ask the patient to lie in the supine position with her legs apart and bent at the knees.

7. Inspect the vulva for vulvitis (red skin), warts, herpes/ulcers, blood or discharge. Genital prolapse can be assessed by gently separating the labia and inspecting the vagina while the patient bears down (Valsalva manoeuvre).

8. Reassuring the patient when things are normal can put the patient at ease and help build a good rapport.

9. Although patients will have some natural lubrication, using water or KY jelly to lubricate the speculum can make the procedure more comfortable for the woman, especially as many women are nervous and find it difficult to relax.

10. Use the non-dominant hand to part the labia, fully exposing the vaginal entrance so you can see where you need to pass the speculum.

11. Warn the patient when you are about to insert the speculum so she can be prepared. Remind her to relax her muscles for you. "Relax your muscles for me I'm going to insert the speculum now."

12. Insert the speculum rotated at 45° so the handle is pointing to the side with the speculum angled slightly downwards. Follow the posterior wall whilst turning the speculum to the horizontal position as you advance, the handle will now be at the top. Advance fully until the end of the speculum is almost level with the perineum. If you do not advance fully it will make it difficult for the cervix to come into view when you open the speculum. Warn the patient that they will feel pressure on the bladder as you open the speculum, but to relax as much as possible.

13. Hold the speculum in position whilst opening the jaws, keep opening it wider until the cervix appears, then fix the speculum.

14. Observe the cervix and vaginal walls for lesions or discharge, which may indicate an abnormality.

15. Take the brush, place the tip into the endocervical canal and turn 5 full rotations in a clockwise direction. Remove the tip of the brush and place into a LABELLED pot and seal.

16. Withdraw the speculum slightly visualizing the cervix till clear (it will hurt if you don't do this and you trap the cervix). Loosen the speculum and allow the jaws to fall together. Continue to withdraw while rotating the speculum onto its side avoiding contact with the anterior structures.

17. The bimanual examination of the pelvis is done after the smear because it can cause trauma, which can ruin the smear sample. It involves palpating the vagina, cervix, uterus and adenexa. Always explain to the patient before proceeding.

18,19. Lubricate the index and middle fingers of your dominant hand.
Part the labia and insert your lubricated index and middle fingers into the vagina following the posterior wall. The thumb should be abducted and the ring and little fingers flexed into the palm. Place your other hand on the patient's abdomen.

20. Feel the position of the cervix, noting its shape, size, mobility and consistency. The cervix normally feels like the tip of your nose, but after pregnancy it feels more like your lips. Check for cervical excitation by gently moving the cervix from side to side. This is very painful if infection is present. Look at the patient's face for signs of discomfort.

21. Palpate the uterus: Put your fingers in the posterior fornix and with your other hand on the patient's abdomen push down towards the hand in the vagina using the palmar surface of your hand to palpate the uterine fundus. Note the size, position, consistency, mobility and tenderness. A normal uterus is the size of a small orange, firm, with a smooth surface. It is freely movable and non-tender. Examine the adnexal structures. Pull back the vaginal hand to clear the cervix. Reposition into the right fornix, palm up. Sweep the right ovary downward with the abdominal hand, 4 cm medial to the iliac crest. Gently trap the ovary between the fingers of both hands (this is not always   possible). Take note of its size and shape. A normal ovary is 2x2cm, almond shaped structure, which is highly mobile and tender to palpation.   Pull back and repeat on the left side. If a mass is found, is it separate from the uterus? Palpate the Pouch of Douglas (behind the cervix): the uterosacral ligaments should be palpable. Are they even? Is there a mass?

22) Thank the patient and allow them to dress in privacy. Always wash your hands to redu ce the risk of cross-infection.

TOP TIPS

ANTENATAL OBSTETRICS EXAMINATION

Look at the woman's general appearance, does she look well? Record her weight, height and temperature. Note whether she has any oedema of the ankles/ sacrum or any signs of anaemia?

The latest NICE guidelines do not recommend routine examination of the chest, breasts and cardiovascular system. Instead a brief enquiry of symptoms and past history relevant to these systems should be made.

Check the blood pressure and perform a dipstick urinalysis. If the blood pressure is raised and/or if there is proteinuria – ask about headaches and palpate for epigastric tenderness. These are signs of pre-eclampsia. Do a fundoscopy if the blood pressure is raised. Also check reflexes for clonus if BP is raised.

Position - Lie the patient as flat as possible, the semiprone position or left lateral tilt is used to avoid aortocaval compression later in pregnancy.

Expose the patient from just below breasts to symphysis pubis.

Inspect the abdomen for size, Striae gravidarum, linea nigra and scars particularly suprapubic scars. Fetal movements may be seen later in pregnancy.

The uterus is normally palpable abdominally at 12 weeks. Palpation should be purposeful and firm but gentle. At < 24 weeks the abdomen is palpated to estimate dates. > 24 weeks, to assess the fetal size and liquor volume (indicators of foetal wellbeing and presence of multiple pregnancy) and greater than 36 weeks to check the lie (transverse or longitudinal), presentation and engagement of the presenting part. After 20 weeks, the symphysis-fundal height (SFH) = the gestation +/- 2cm for a normal singleton pregnancy. A raised SFH may be due to incorrect dates, multiple pregnancy, diabetes, polyhydramnios. A reduced SFH may be due to Intrauterine growth retardation (IUGR), oligohydramnios, incorrect dates.

Presentation refers to the part that occupies the lower segment. It is either cephalic (head descending first) or breech (bottom / feet first). To assess this have your hands facing the pelvis. Press the fingers of both hands down firmly, just above the symphysis pubis. The engagement of the head is described as 'fifths' palpable. If only two-fifths of the baby's head is palpable above the symphisis pubis,the other 3/5 must be engaged. If more than 2/5 is palpable then the head is not yet engaged.

Also feel for any uterine tenderness.

Auscultate for the fetal heart rate over the fetus's anterior shoulder with either a Doppler ultrasound or a Pinard stethoscope. This is usually found between the head and the umbilicus. Normally the fetal heart rate is between 110-160 beats per minute and resembles the loud ticking of a watch (when auscultated with a Pinard stethoscope).

Vaginal examination is not a routine part of antenatal examination unless labour is suspected or is to be induced.

Screening Tests (routinely offered)

Infections

Rubella
Syphilis
Hepatitis B
HIV

Fetal Anomalies

Down syndrome   β-hCG
                       PAPP-A (Pregnancy associated plasma protein A)
                       α-fetoprotein (AFP)
                       Serum unconjugated oestriol
                       Serum Inhibin-A
                       NT (nuchal translucency) measurement

Neural tube defects   Serum α-fetoprotein (AFP)

Haematological disorders

Anaemia
Hamoglobinopathies (thalassaemia, sickle cell)
Red cell alloantibodies and prophylactic anti-D

PAEDIATRICS

NEONATAL EXAMINATION

- Note birth weight, gestational age and centile.
- Aim is to exclude congenital abnormalities and infection.

		Not Attempted	Attempted inadequate	Attempt adequate
1.	Introduces self to parents, explains role and gains consent	0	1	2
2.	Wash hands and fully undresses infant	0	1	2
3.	Completes a general inspection of the infant	0	1	2
4.	Correctly examines the head and neck including sutures and the fontenelles	0	1	2
5.	Examines the mouth and palate	0	1	2
6.	Auscultates the lungs	0	1	2
7.	Examines the cardiovascular system	0	1	2
8.	Palpates the abdomen	0	1	2
9.	Examines external genitalia and anus	0	1	2
10.	Examines the neurological system and primitive reflexes			
11.	Checks spine	0	1	2
12.	Check for congenital dislocation of the hips	0	1	2
13.	Reassure the parents if everything is normal	0	1	2
14.	Washes hands	0	1	2

1) It is polite to introduce yourself, explain why you are there and get verbal consent from the parents.

2) Fully undress the infants including the nappy.

3) General inspection/examination
Look at the colour of the child comment on pallor/jaundice/cyanosis.
Check the tongue for central cyanosis. Jaundice within 24hrs of birth is usually pathological and requires further investigation.

Look for features of dysmorphism, look at the facies (downs syndrome is the most common) and look for a single palmer crease.

Observe for any signs of trauma (may be present after instrumental delivery).

Check the skin for any birthmarks or rashes. Preterm babies may have thin skin.

Common lesions:

- "Stork mark" – very common; flat, red macules, on forehead and nape of neck; those around the eyes usually resolve.
- Capillary haemangioma ("port wine stain") - red to purple flat lesion; can occur anywhere, do not disappear; if unilateral especially on face, can have special significance – may be associated with intra-cranial haemangioma.
- Cavernous haemangioma ("strawberry naevus") may or may not be present at birth as a raised red/purple birthmark. These increase in size over the first few months of life and then slowly regress. They may need intervention depending on their site eg those in the region of the eye if they occlude vision.
- Mongolian spots – blue discolouration on the buttocks and lumbosacral areas (more common in darker skinned babies).
- Milia - plugged sweat glands causing red spots on face and nose.
- Erythema toxicum common on day 2-3 – red popular lesions on trunk

Observe infants behaviour (are they active and happy?).
Feel the temperature of the infant.
Count fingers and toes! (Syndactyly – fingers bound together. Polydactyly – extra digit).
Look for clubbed feet (turned in), if they are difficult to correct with pressure there may be structural rather than positional talipes.

4) Head
Inspect for bruises, cuts, and presence of hair.
Comment on the shape. Caput succedaneum is swelling of part of the head due to pressure from delivery on presenting part (cone head!)
Moulding (overriding of cranial bones) is normal following delivery it normally resolves within 5 days.
Measure the circumference using a paper tape measure (measures brain size) usually 33-38cm.
Check the mobility of suture lines. The saggital suture is often separated and the coronal sutures may be overriding. Craniosynostosis is early suture closing.

The anterior and posterior fontanelles are normally flat and soft but not sunken. The size of the fontanelle varies. If the fontanelle is tense when the baby is not crying, consider raised intracranial pressure. A cranial ultrasound should be done to exclude hydrocephalus. Tense fontanelles are also a late sign of meningitis.

Check the shape and position of the **ears;** low set ears may be a sign of dysmorphism; ear malformations including pre-auricular skin tags or pits may be associated with genitourinary anomalies. Check the range of rotation of the head to each side. Observe the neck for webbing or masses.

Check the baby's **eyes** in a darkened room using an ophthalmoscope to elicit the red reflex. Look for congenital cataracts. Check pupil constriction to light.
5) Mouth inspect and palpate the palate using your little finger to check for cleft palate and other deformities (can also check sucking reflex at the same time).

6) Respiratory system
Observe breathing and chest wall movements for signs of respiratory distress. Auscultate the lungs and listen for any noisy breathing / grunting. Periodic breathing is common in early newborn period, especially in pre-term babies.

7) Cardiovascular system

Feel for the apex and auscultate heart, listening for any murmurs or added sounds. The normal heart rate in baby's is110-150 bpm. Check capillary refill over the sternum < 4 seconds is normal.

Palpate the femoral pulses. The pulse pressure is decreased in coarctation of the aorta and increased in patent ductus arteriosus. Check the pulses are equal and for radial-femoral delay.

8) Palpate abdomen – for organs and any masses. It is normal to be able to palpate a soft liver edge, 1 cm below the costal margin, in the neonate; the spleen tip may be palpable, as may the kidneys. Careful inspection of umbilicus should be done looking for, signs of infection, bleeding, discharge, herniation. Auscultate for bowel sounds.

9) Inspect genitalia and anus

Boys:
Check penis size > 2.5cm.
Check for phimosis (common, foreskin not fully retracted, may not retract in many for years).
Look at position of urethra. (Hypospadias is where the urethra opens on underside of the penis, and often needs correcting).
Confirm presence of testis in scrotum (start from internal ring)
Check for scrotal hernias.

Girls:
Check the labia majora and minora for enlargement or mucosal tags. Part the labia to check for vaginal fusion. A white vaginal discharge is normal in baby girls.

Anus:
Check anus for patency (opening), position and size of anus. Ask if child has passed meconium within 24-48 hrs of birth (this in itself confirms patency!). Consider Hirschprung's Disease if this has not occurred.

10) Neurological examination

Observing limb movements assesses muscle tone. Look for symmetry of movements. With Erb's palsy you get a decreased motion of the arm.
On turning the baby prone, the baby's head should lift to the horizontal position and the back straightens.
Assess tone further by pulling the infant's arms from a flat position. The head will lag. It is therefore important to provide support for the head as necessary.

Examine primitive reflexes:

Moro reflex (startle reflex) – normally present till 4 months after birth. Hold the infant supine, a few inches above the bed, gently drop infant's head to illicit startle and quickly support it again. The baby should appear startled and throw out arms in abduction then adduction as it relaxes. 2-sided absence suggests brain or spinal cord damage. Unilateral loss may be due to brachial plexus injury or fractured collarbone or other bone in the arm. A moro reflex in an older child is abnormal. When the infant is crying it is sometimes not possible to elicit a normal Moro reflex. NB Leave this towards end of examination as it is upsetting for the baby.
Rooting reflex touch newborn on either cheek, the baby will turn to find the breast.
Sucking reflex the baby should suck when a finger or object is placed into its mouth.

Palmar and plantar grasp reflexes – are demonstrated by stimulating the palm and sole respectively.

11) Spine
Inspect back and spine with baby prone. Feel for any abnormalities and look for midline defects of the skin.

12) Hips check for developmental dysplasia of the hips (leave this till last as it is uncomfortable and baby will most likely cry making the rest of your examination more difficult). This is done using **Barlow's** and **Ortolani's** tests.
Recognition in the early neonatal period is essential for proper treatment.

13) Reassuring the parents if everything is normal is important to put their minds at ease.

14) Wash hands.

PAEDIATRIC HISTORY

		Not Attempted	Attempted inadequate	Attempted adequate
1.	Introduces self, explains role and obtains consent	0	1	2
2.	Asks about presenting complaint and history of presenting complaint	0	1	2
3.	Asks about the pregnancy, delivery and neonatal period	0	1	2
4.	Asks about child's development and appropriate milestones	0	1	2
5.	Asks about child's growth?	0	1	2
6.	Checks if immunisations are up to date?	0	1	2
7.	Asks about the Past Medical History	0	1	2
8.	Asks social history	0	1	2
9.	Asks family history	0	1	2
10.	Reviews systems enquiry	0	1	2
11.	Asks drug history and allergies	0	1	2
12.	Demonstrates a good standard of communication	0	1	2

1) Introduces self to the child and parents. For a younger child verbal consent from the parents is needed before taking the history. Don't forget to address questions to the child when appropriate

2) Ask about why they are here, specifically, what prompted them to come to the doctor?

Let the parents and child recount the presenting complaint in their own words and at their own pace.

Onset (sudden / gradual)? Duration? History of Presenting Complaint (have they ever had anything like this before?) Is it getting better or worse? Is it there all the time or does it come and go? Does anything make it relieve or aggravate it?

Ask when was your child last well?

It may be helpful to ask the parents what their concerns are.

3) Find out about the Pregnancy & Delivery
- Planned/unplanned/adopted/assisted pregnancy (IVF). Extreme discretion and sensitivity are needed to ask these questions if information not volunteered and not normally asked in the first instance – if children adopted parents will usually volunteer.
- Normal scans during pregnancy?
- Mode of delivery – vaginal delivery, spontaneous or induced, if c-section was it emergency or elective and why?
- Any resuscitation needed at birth?
- SCBU admissions after birth
- Birth weight

- Neonatal jaundice
- Breast fed or bottle fed?

4) Ask if there are any concerns about the child's vision, hearing or development?
How are they doing at school, regarding work and behaviour? Do they like school?
Do they have friends at school?
Are there any problems with bladder and bowel control?
Do they have problems sleeping?
Development screen for children under 5 yrs (or over 5s if there are development problems).

DEVELOPMENTAL MILESTONES
Smiling by 6 weeks
Sit unsupported by 9 months
Turns to sound 6 months
First words by 18 months
Walking by 18-months
Links 2 words in mini-sentences by 3 years.

5) Any problems with their growth? Are they smaller or larger than their friends?
Review their growth records in Red Book if available.
6) Are their immunisations up to date?
Review their immunisation record in Red Book if available. Current immunisation guidelines are given below.
7) Do they see their GP for anything regularly?
Ask about previous illnesses, hospital admissions, accidents, injuries or operations?
8)Social History involves checking relevant information about the family, their home and the community.
Ask about housing (rented or owned / house or flat)?
Ask who's at home
Are their any pets at home?
Ask parent's occupations?
Ever involved with social services? (be tactful).
Ask whether the parents smoke or use any illicit drugs? If so, do they smoke in the home?
Taking a good social history is vital as many childhood illnesses are affected by adult problems e.g. poverty, damp housing, poor diet, unstable partnerships, psychiatric disorders, parental illness and alcohol/drug abuse.
9) Family history (mum, dad, brothers and sisters). Is there consanguinity? Do d
Does anyone in the family suffer from any similar problems or serious medical conditions?
10) Systems examination – ask about general health. Is the child normally lively and active?

Respiratory - breathing difficulties, cough, wheeze, cyanosis (has the child ever gone blue?)
Cardiovascular – murmurs, cyanosis, breathlessness (especially when feeding)
Nutrition In infants ask if the child is breastfed and whether there are any problems with feeding? Is the child satisfied by their feeds or are the parents having to give top up's. How much milk does the child take during one sitting and how often are they feeding? If the child is taking formula milk, which type?
For a child of 6months ask whether they are on solids?
Does the child have any special dietary requirements?

Gastrointestinal – Vomiting, diarrhoea, constipation, abdominal pain, jaundice.
Renal – Urinary frequency, wetting, blood in the urine, urinary tract infections, unexplained fever, periorbital oedema / ascites (swollen eyes and abdomen are clinical features of nephrotic syndrome).
ENT – throat / ear infections
Dermatology – rashes / skin conditions.
Neurological – fits, faints, headaches or abnormal movements.
Rheumatological / orthopaedic – swollen / painful joints or muscles. Broken bones?

11) Ask about current medications and any allergies.

12) Establish a rapport with the family as a whole with occasional playful remarks or actions to the child.

The UK's immunisation schedule (2008)

Age	Diseases against which immunised	Vaccines
Two months old	Diphtheria, tetanus, pertussis (whooping cough), polio and Haemophilus influenzae type b (Hib) Pneumococcal infection	DTaP/IPV/Hib Pneumococcal conjugate vaccine, (PCV)
Three months old	Diphtheria, tetanus, pertussis, polio and Haemophilus influenzae type b (Hib) Meningitis C	DTaP/IPV/Hib MenC
Four months old	Diphtheria, tetanus, pertussis, polio and Haemophilus influenzae type b (Hib) Meningitis C Pneumococcal infection	DTaP/IPV/Hib MenC PCV
Around 12 months old	Haemophilus influenza type b (Hib) Meningitis C	Hib/MenC
Around 13 months old	Measles, mumps and rubella Pneumococcal infection	MMR PCV
Three years and four months or soon after	Diphtheria, tetanus, pertussis and polio Measles, mumps and rubella	DTaP/IPV or dTaP/IPV MMR
Thirteeen to eighteen years old	Diphtheria, tetanus, polio	Td/IPV
Thirteen to eighteen years old (from September 2008 - girls only)	Human papilloma virus (HPV) - increases the risk of cervical cancer	HPV

In addition, some babies in high-risk groups are given a BCG immunisation for protection against tuberculosis shortly after they are born. Higher risk infants may also receive immunisation against Hepatitis B.
http://www.direct.gov.uk/en/Parents/Yourchildshealthandsafety/YourChildsHealth/DG_10026138

289

References and suggested reading

- Kumar P, Clark M (eds). *Clinical medicine.* Fourth edition (1999). W.B. Saunders.

- Munro JF, Campbell IW (eds). *Macleod's clinical examination.* Tenth edition (2000). Churchill Livingstone.

- Talley NJ, O'Connor S. *Clinical examination. A systematic guide to physical diagnosis.* Fourth edition (2001). Blackwell Science.

- Epstein O, Perkin DG, de Bono DP, Cookson J. *Pocket guide to clinical examination.* Second edition (1997). Mosby.

- Clayden. G, Lissauer. T. Illustrated Textbook Of Paediatrics.2nd edition. 2001. Mosby.

- Impey. L. Obstetrics & Gunaecology. 2nd edition. 2004. Blackwell Publishing.

- Longmore. M, Rajagopalan. S.R, Wilkinson. I,B. Oxford Handbook Of Clinical Medicine. 6th edition. 2004. Oxford University Press.